Strong Like Me

Understanding CANCER

A Gentle Picture Book About Cancer and Treatment for Young Children

To: ____________________

From: ____________________

Written by Dr. Fei Zheng-Ward

Illustrated by Buttercup Studio

Identifiers: ISBN 979-8-89318-144-9 (eBook)
ISBN 979-8-89318-219-4 (paperback)
ISBN 979-8-89318-146-3 (hardcover)

All living things are made of teeny-tiny pieces called cells.

Cells are like little building blocks that are much, much smaller than the tip of a pencil.

People have cells.

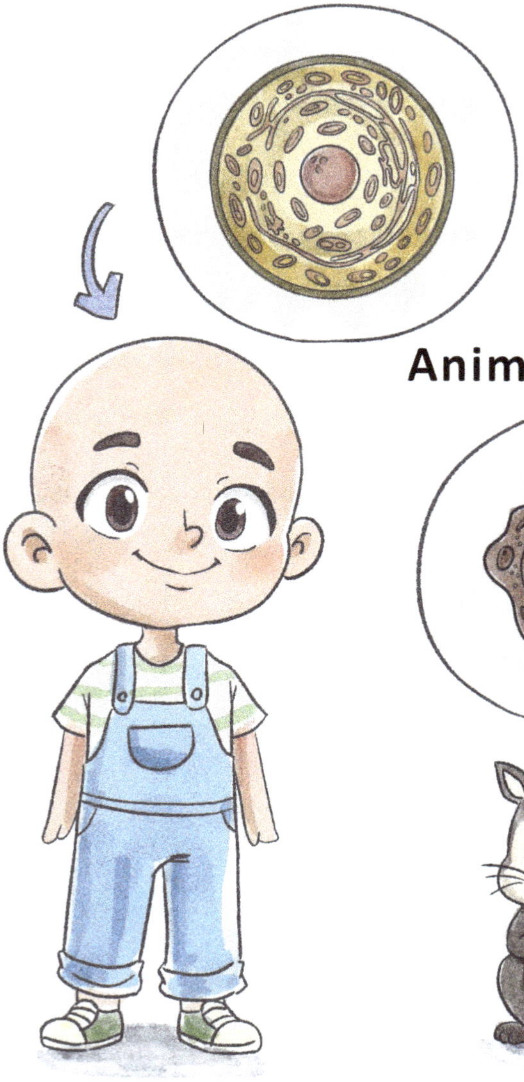

Animals have cells.

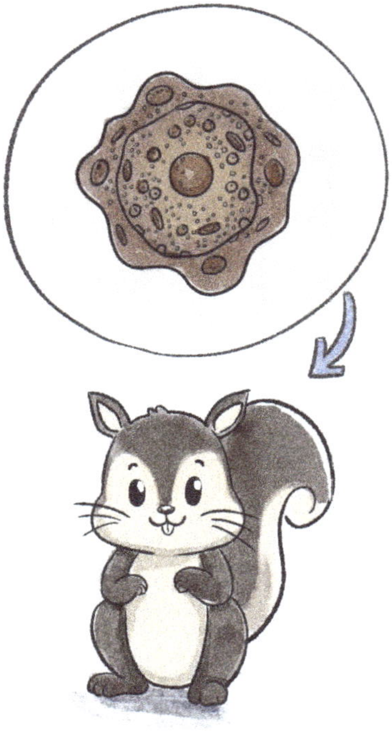

Plants have cells too.

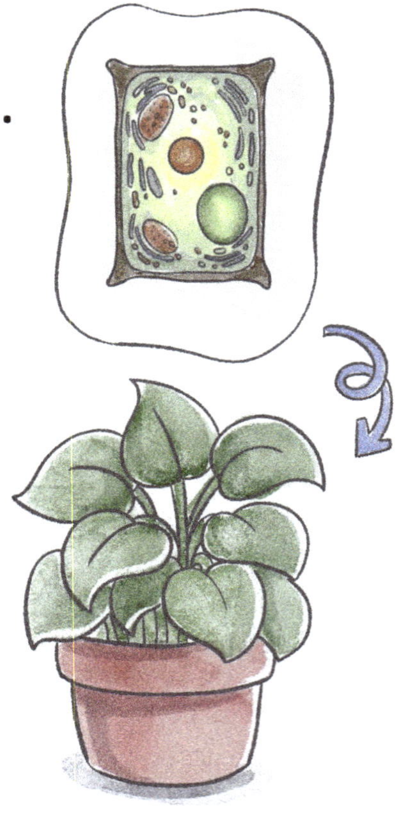

Cells help our bodies grow and heal.

Normal cells know when to grow
and when to stop.

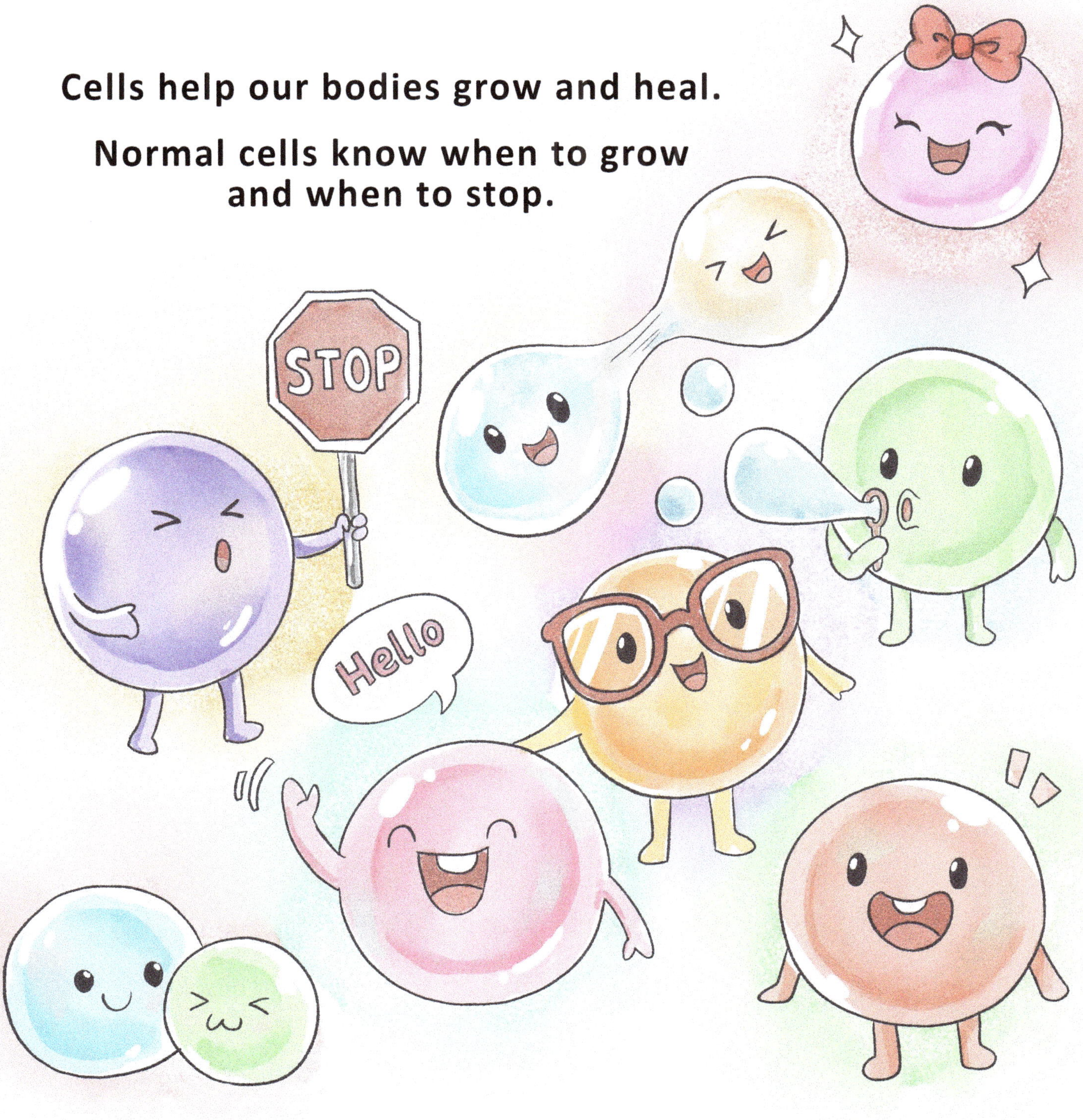

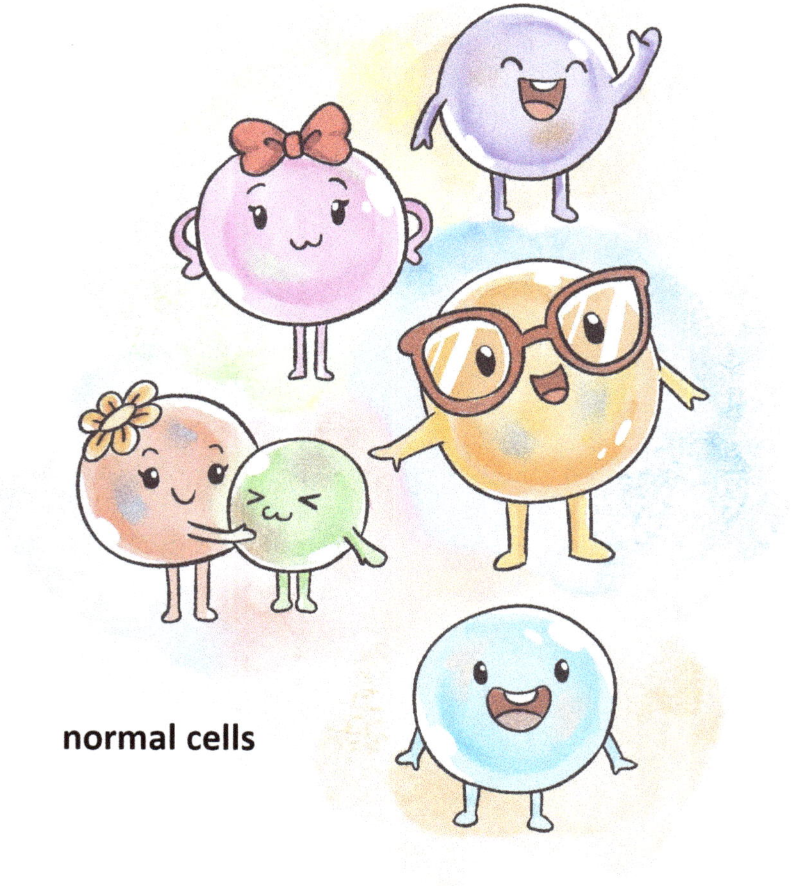

Most of the time, cells do their job.

Sometimes, cells get mixed up
and don't know when to stop growing.

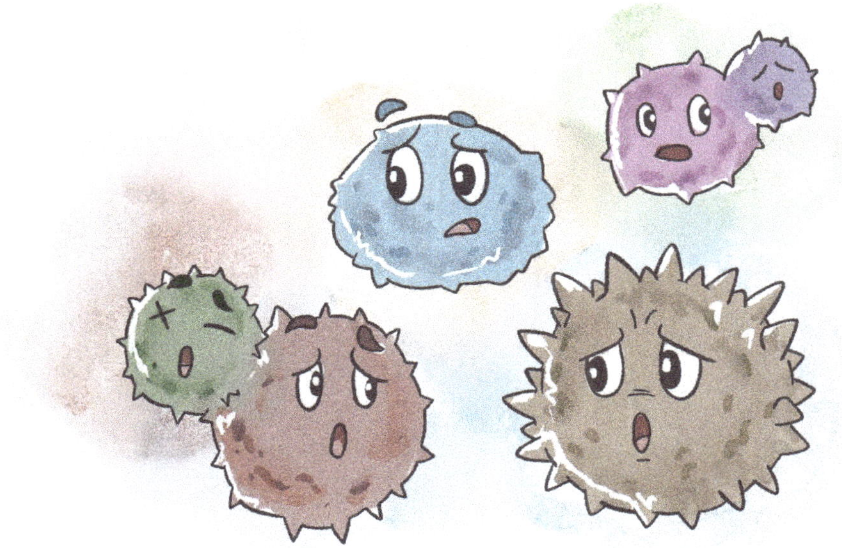

Mixed-up cells don’t help the body.

Cancer is when mixed-up cells make
too many copies of themselves.

Here are some places where cancer can grow.

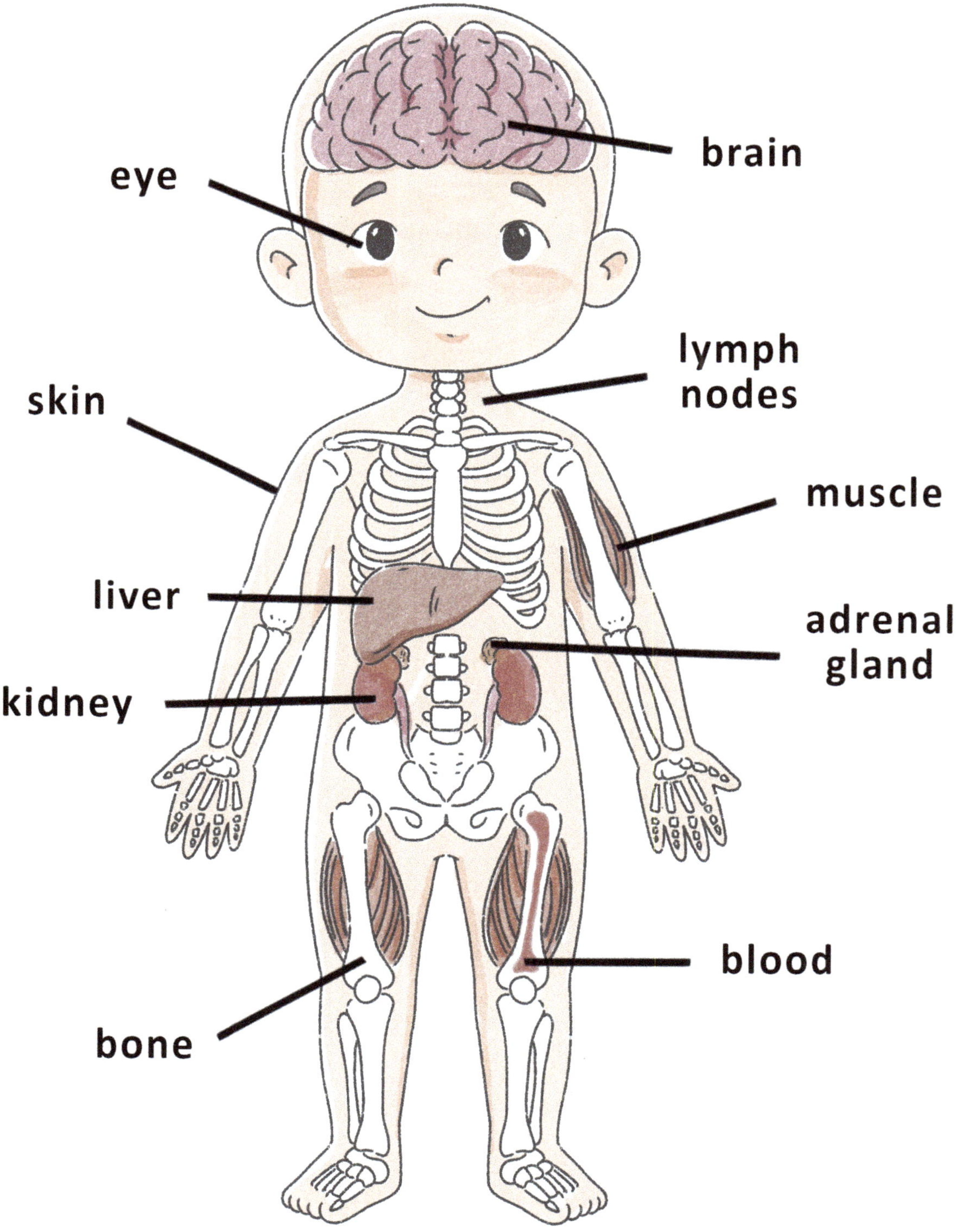

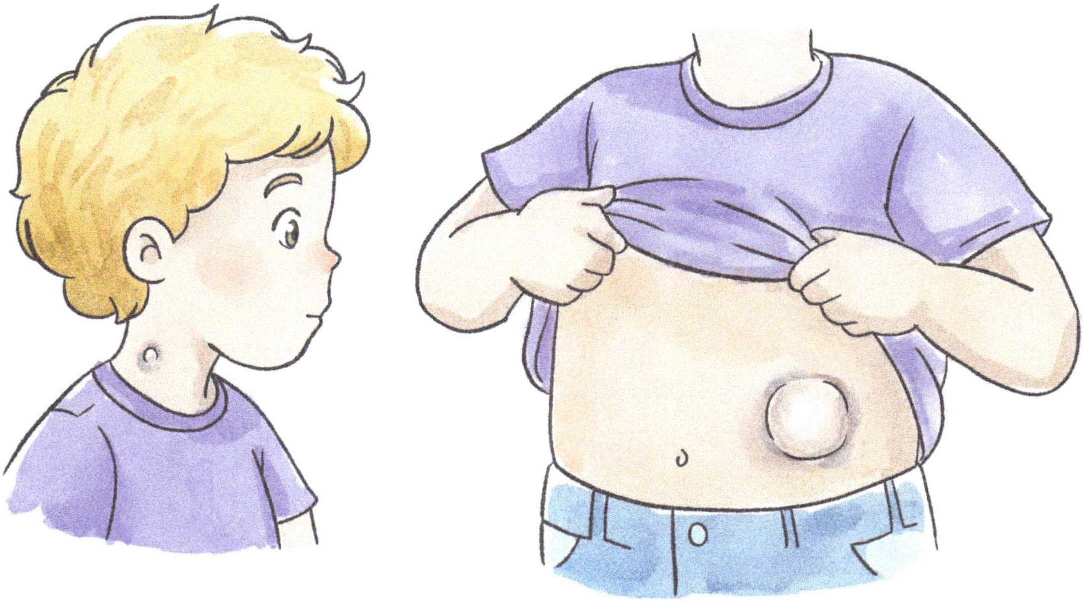

If the cancer is close to the skin or is big enough,
you may feel a bump (called a lump).

Let’s help your body feel calm and strong.

How would you like to help?

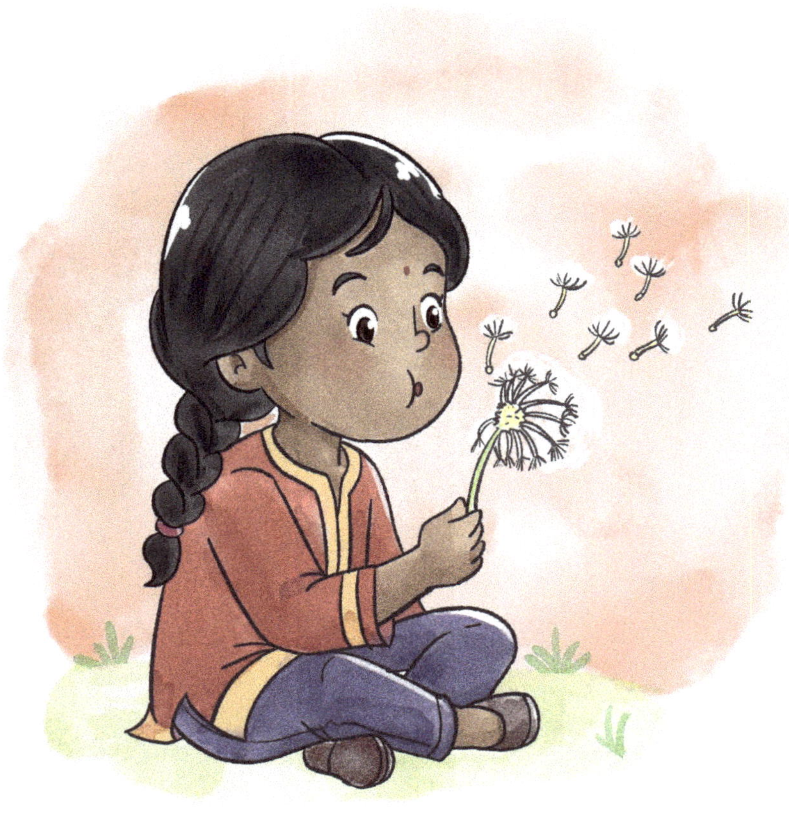

Blow gently like you’re blowing dandelion seeds?

Or pretend you're blowing a big, slow bubble?

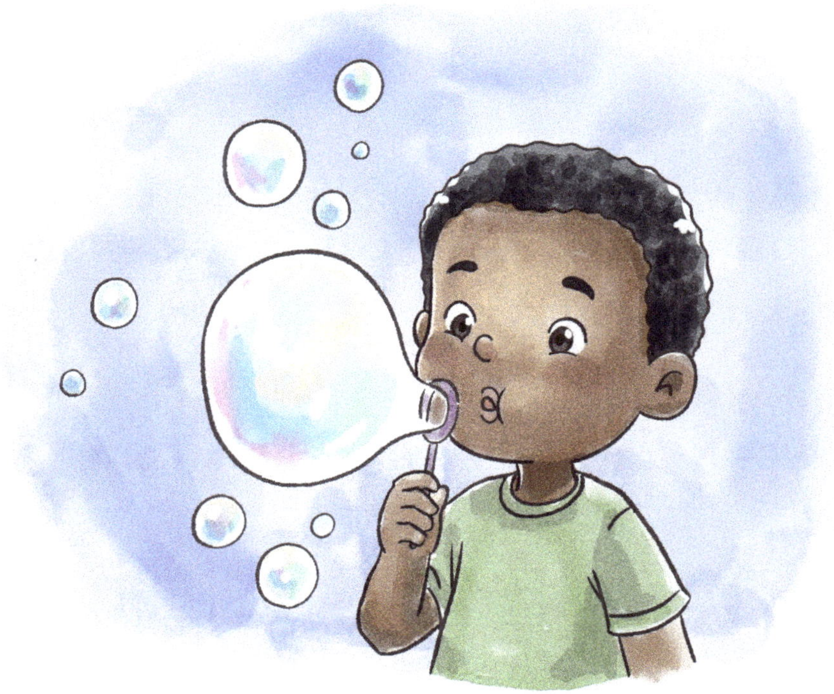

Take a slow breath in...

Now blow softly...

When you blow slowly,
you are helping your body feel calm.

Now imagine the mixed-up cells
floating away and getting smaller.

What creative ideas do you have to help
your body feel calm and strong?

Your body tries hard to stay healthy,
but sometimes it needs help.

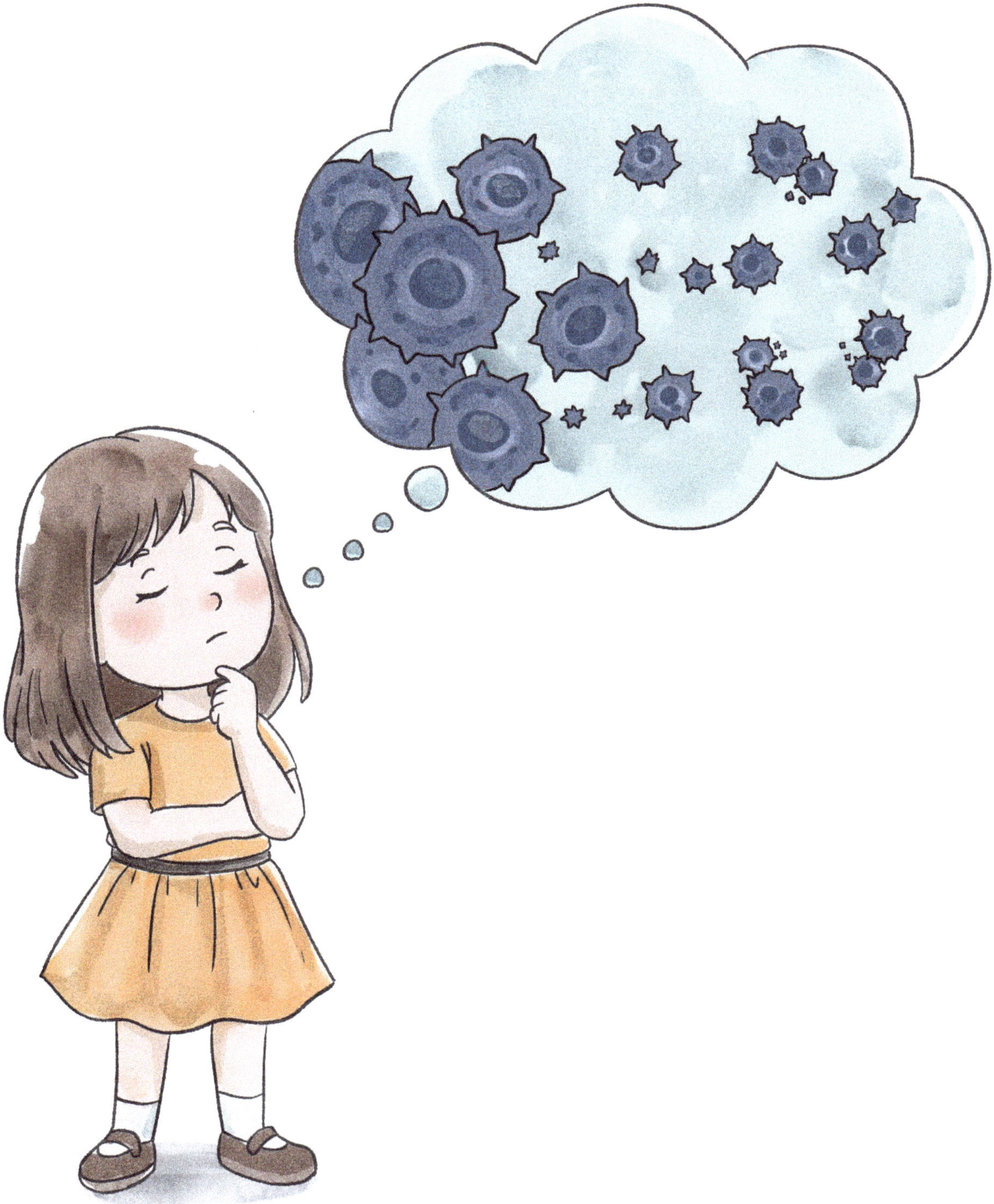

Doctors, nurses, hospital helpers,
and special treatments help remove
the mixed-up cells and help your body heal.

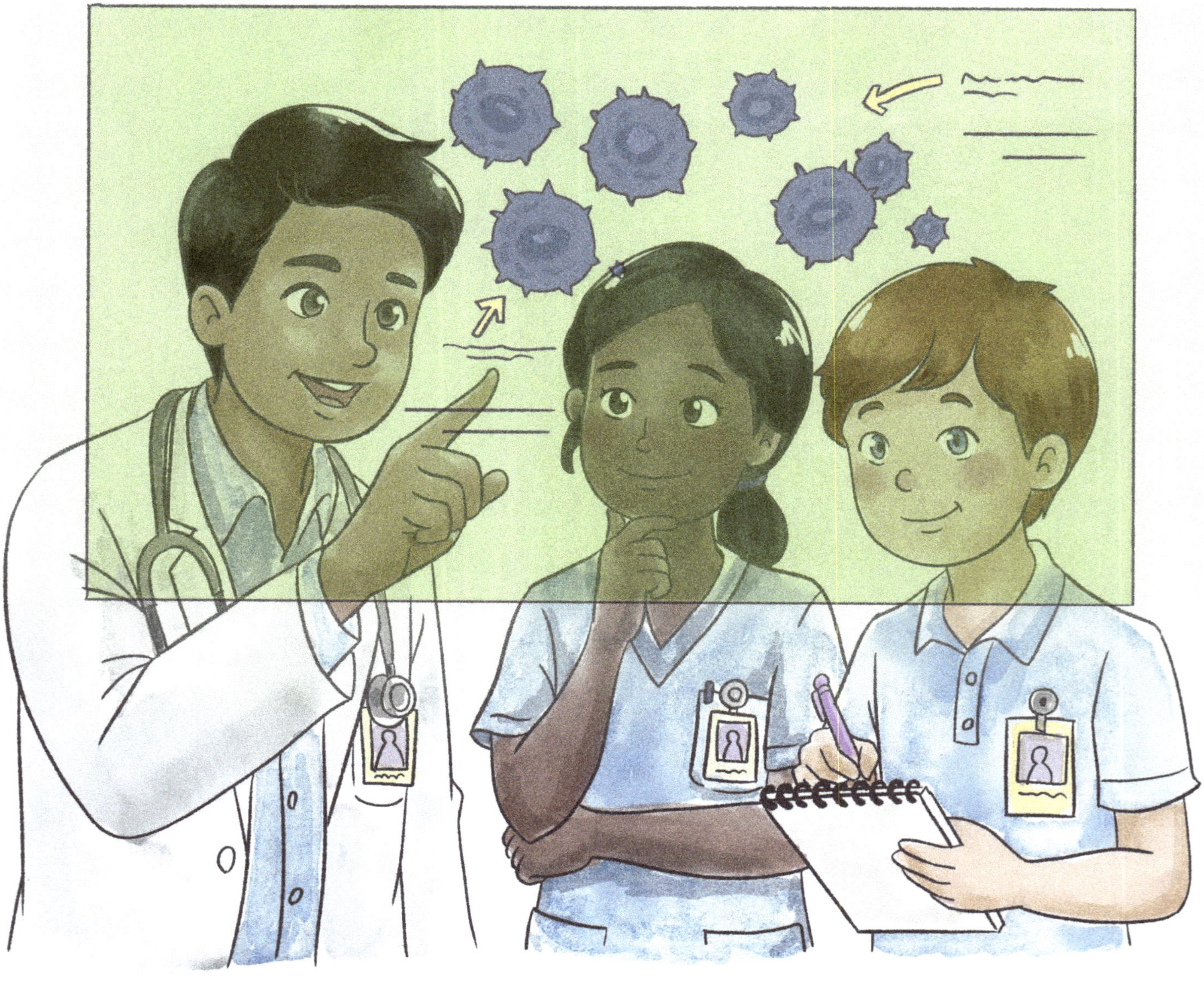

You can help by

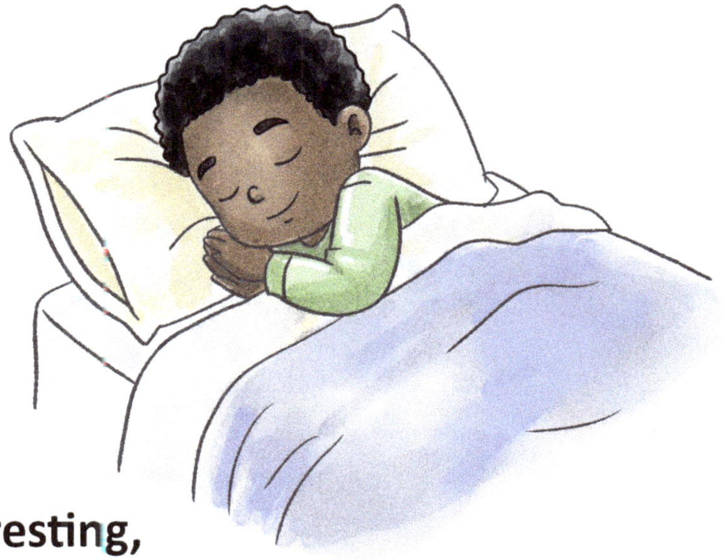

resting,

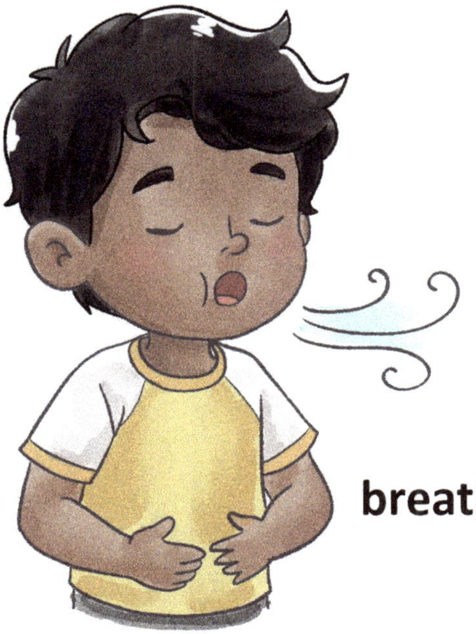

breathing,

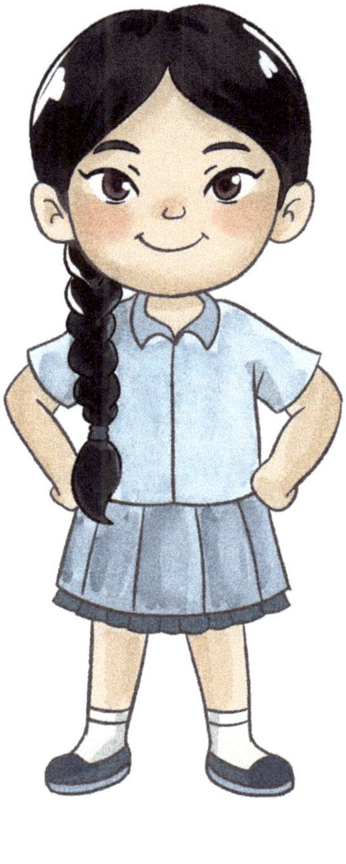

and being
brave.

Doctors help the body by using special treatments such as

1) Medicine called **chemotherapy**
2) Strong, invisible light called **radiation**
3) Taking out the lump (called **surgery**)

Often, more than one kind of treatment is used.

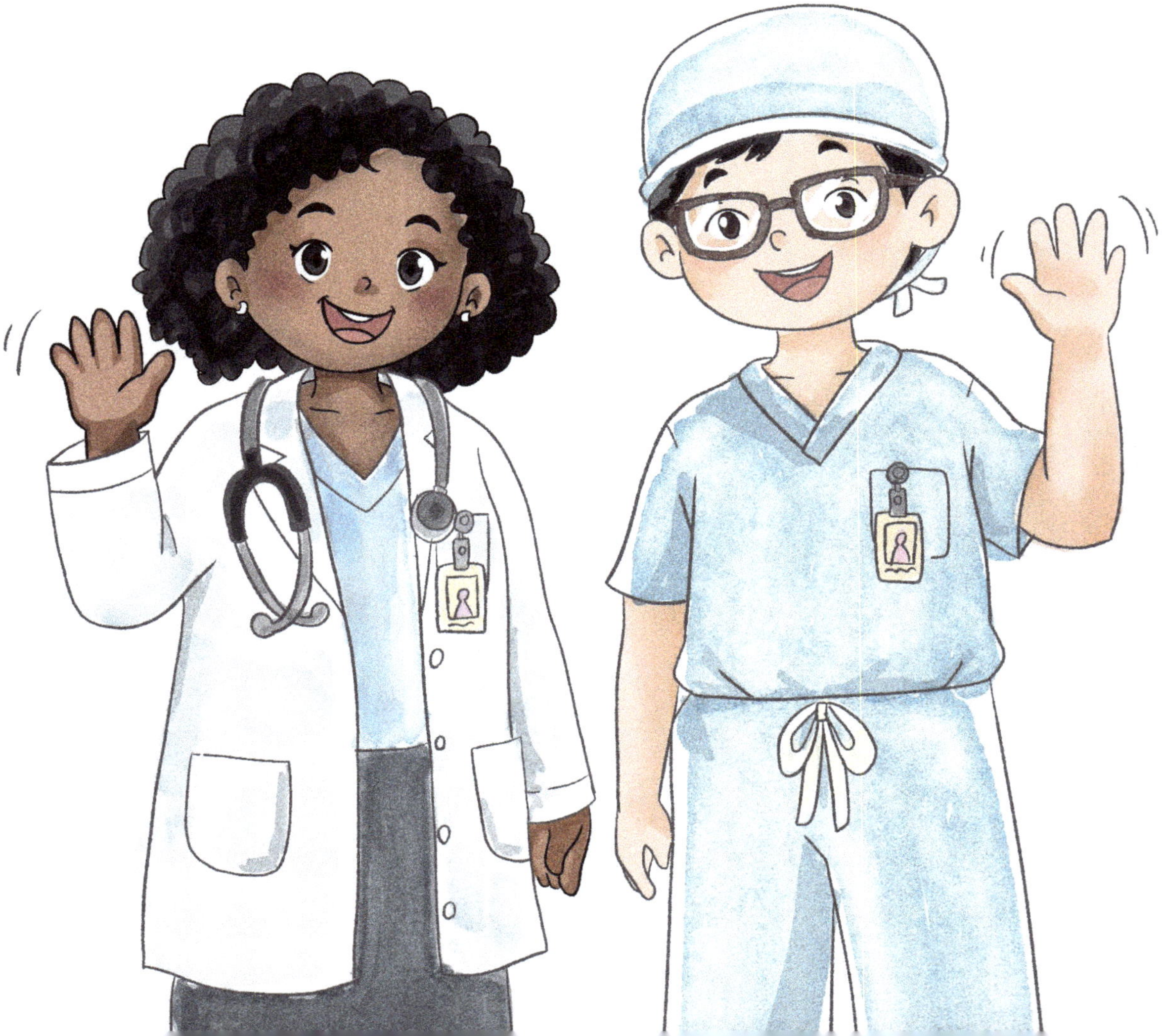

These treatments are made to help you.

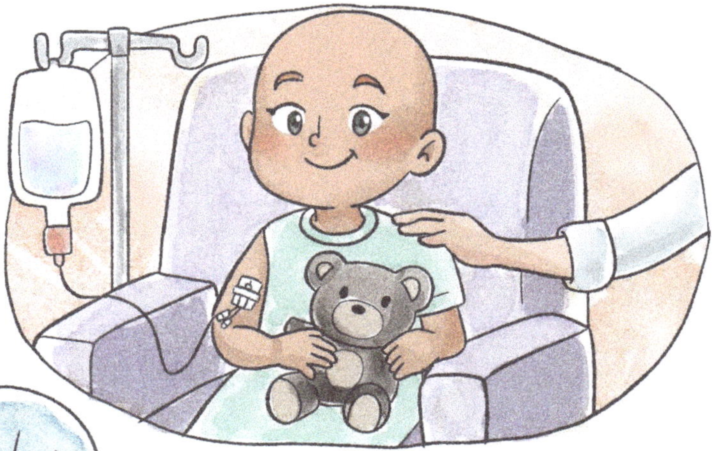

Chemotherapy

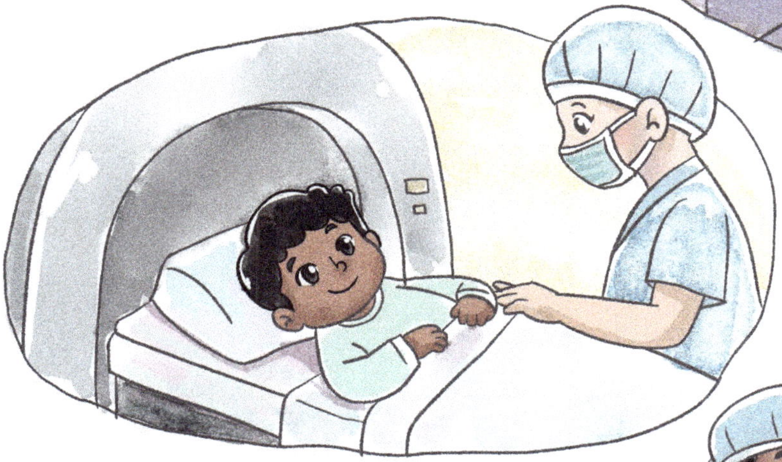

Radiation

Surgery

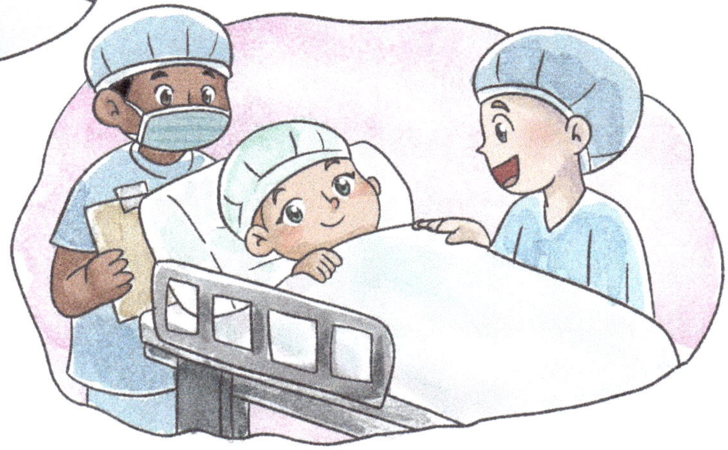

Doctors, nurses, and hospital helpers work together to keep you safe and comfortable.

Chemotherapy is strong medicine that helps chase away mixed-up cells.

The medicine may go into your body through a small button on your chest (called a port).

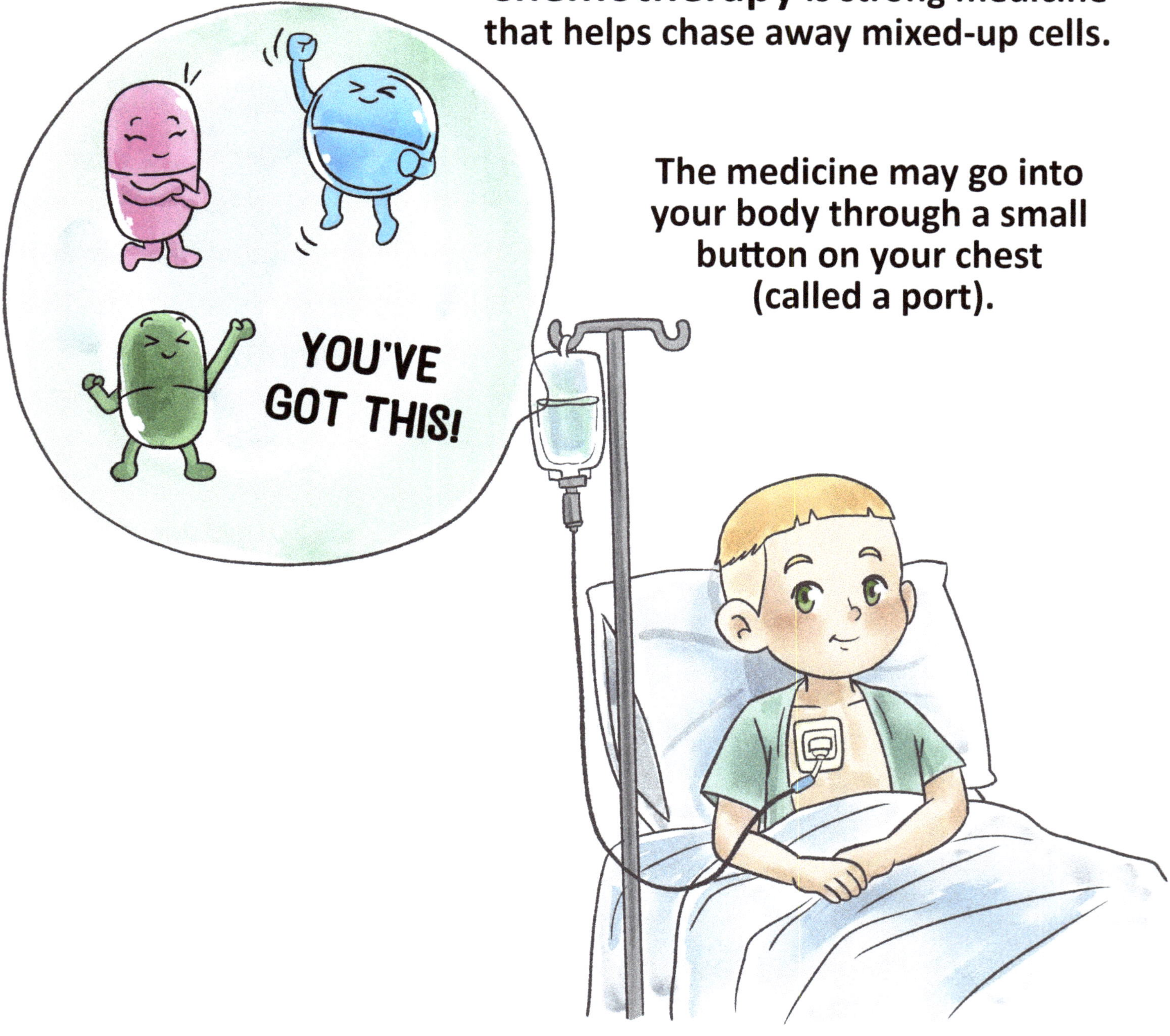

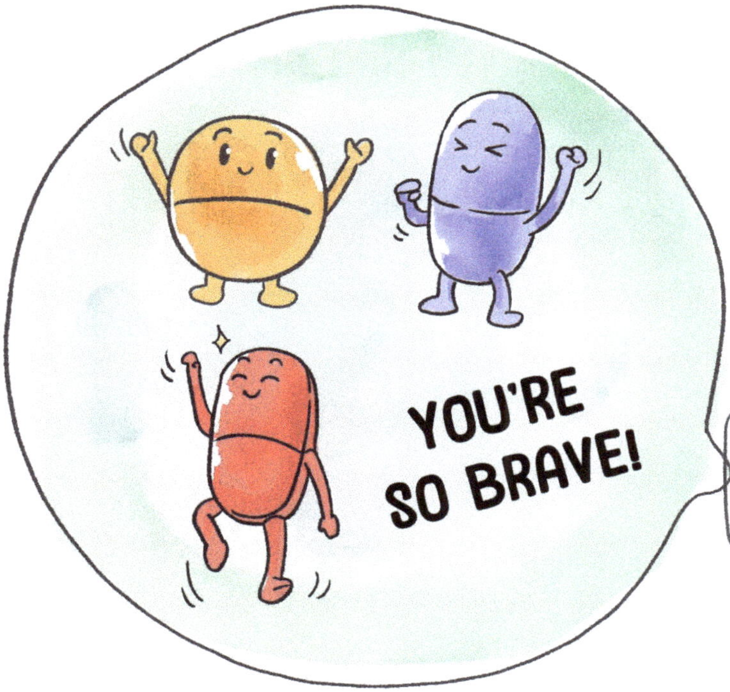

You may feel tired or sick to your tummy.

Clean hands and gentle touches help keep you safe.

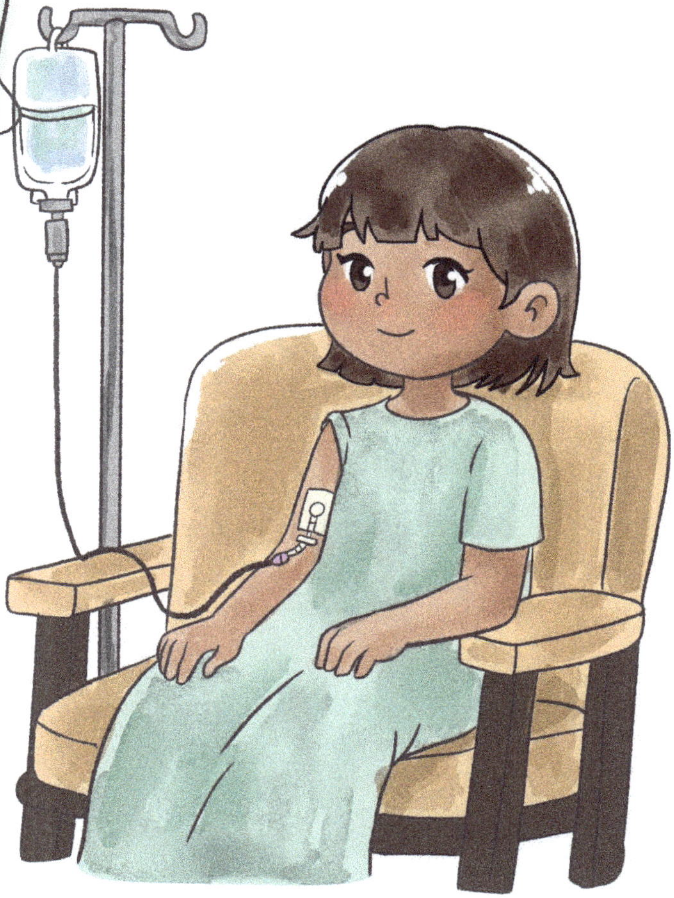

Or it may go through a tiny tube in your arm (called a PICC line).

You, your doctor, and your grown-up will choose the best one for you.

Radiation therapy uses strong, invisible light.
The light also helps chase away mixed-up cells.

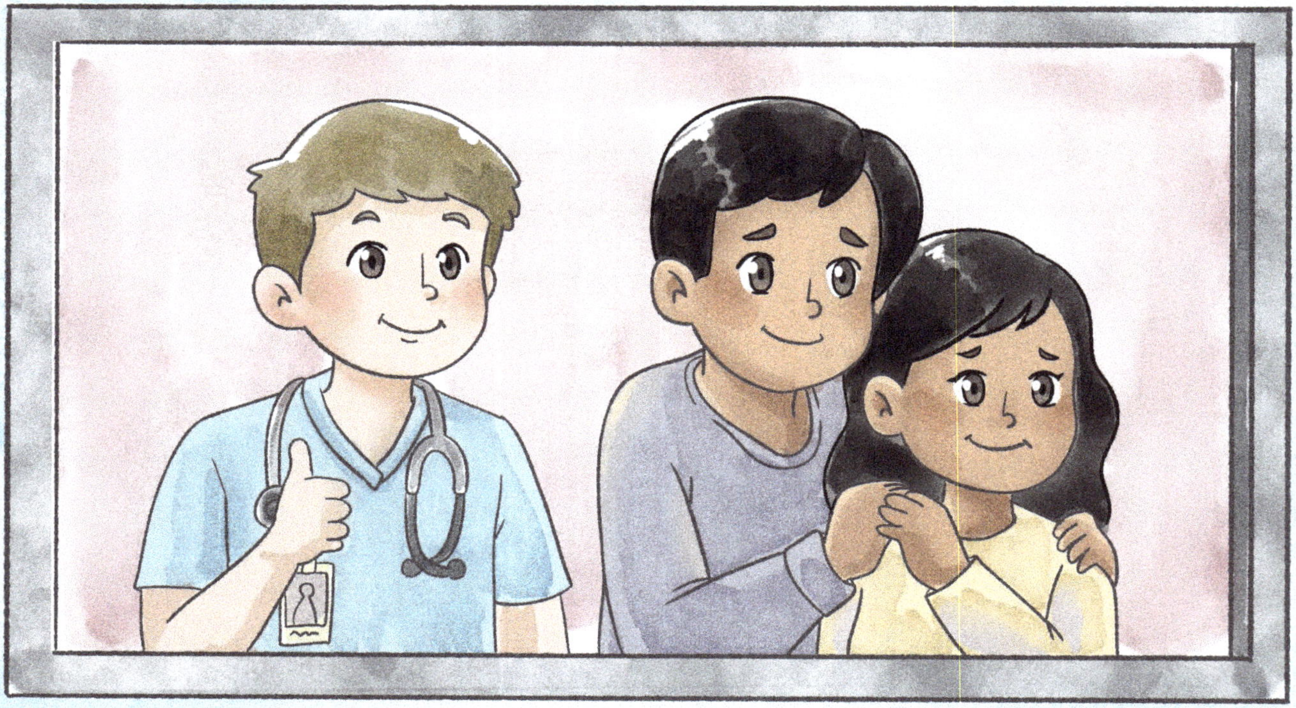

The machine may be big and loud.

But, you cannot see or feel the light.

Lying very still helps a lot.

If staying still is hard, special sleepy medicine can help your body rest.

Your grown-up and hospital helpers are close by, watching and keeping you safe and comfortable.

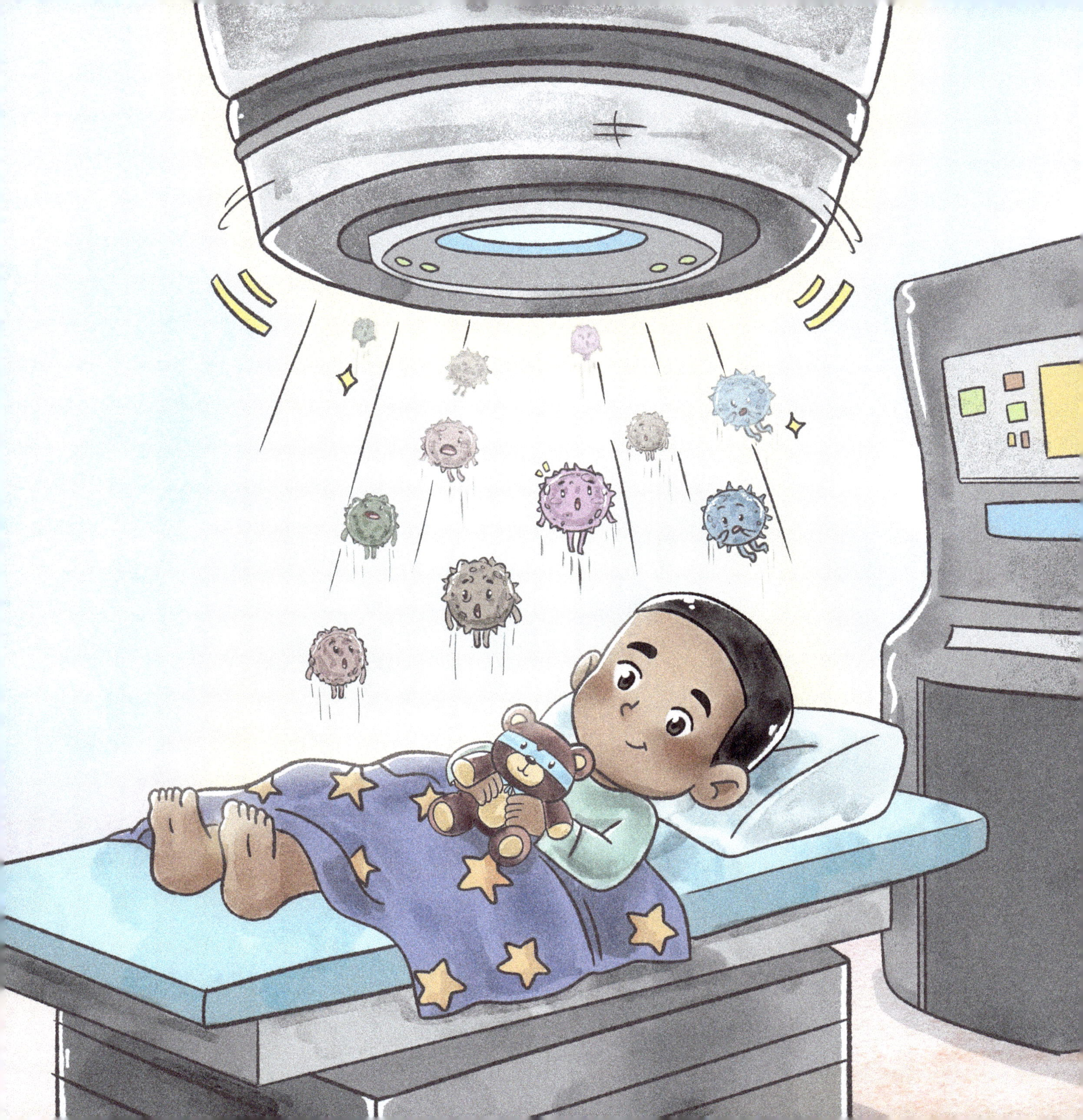

For some cancers, doctors can do **surgery**.

Surgery helps take the cancer out of the body.

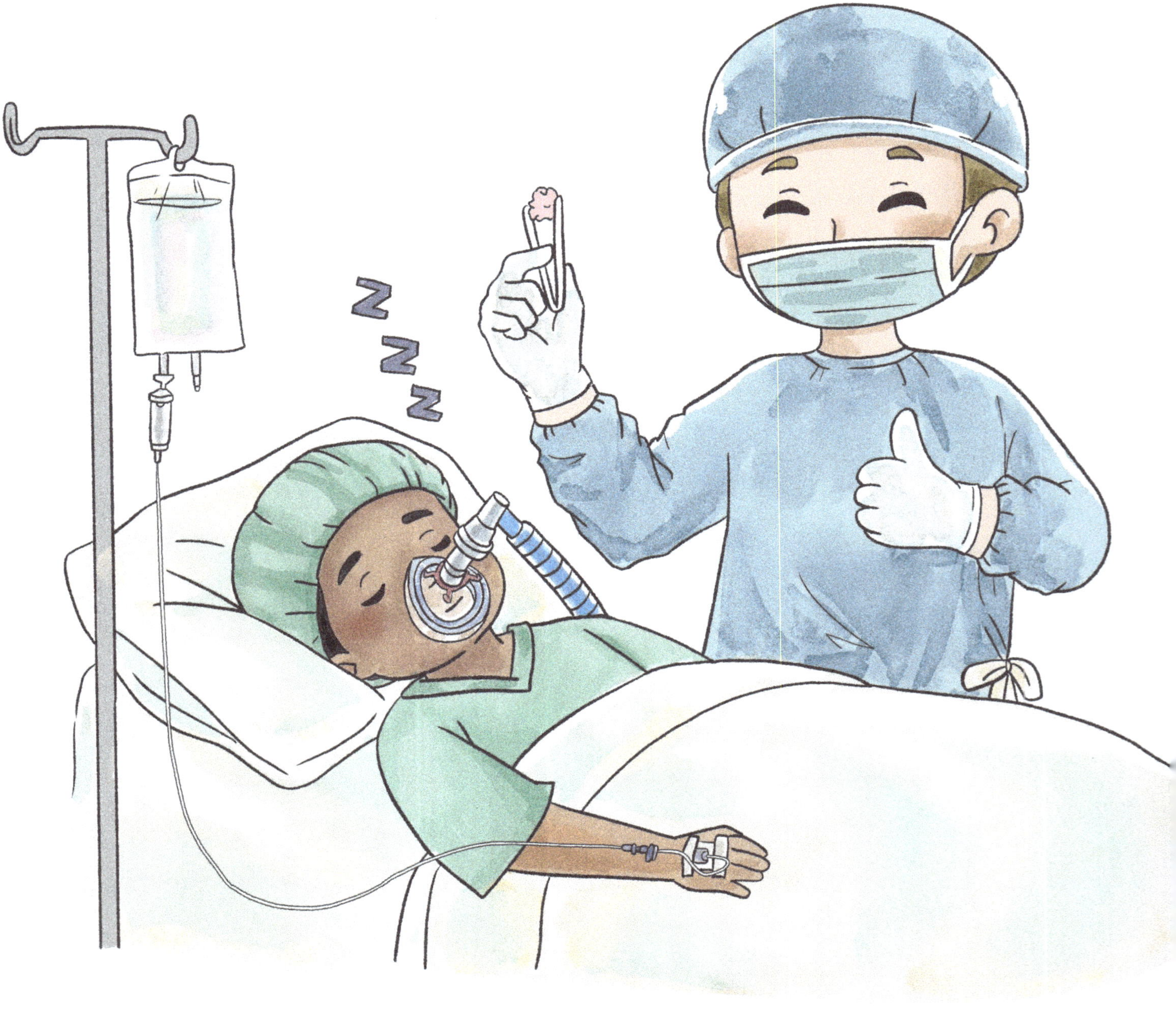

After surgery,
you may feel sore.

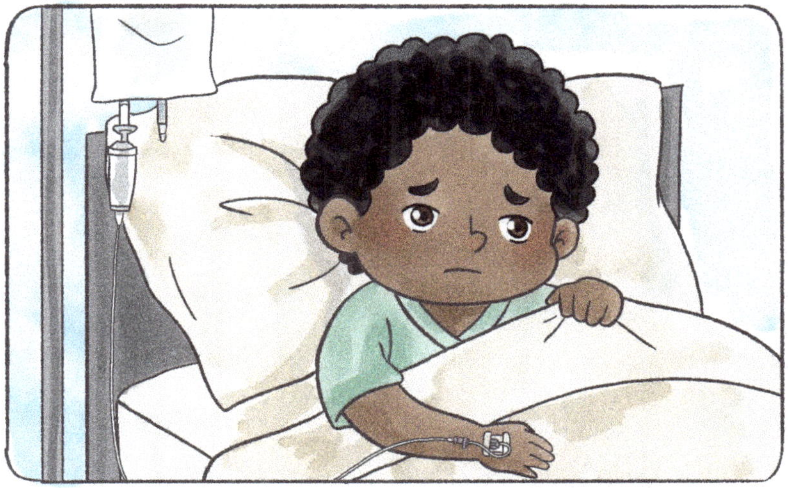

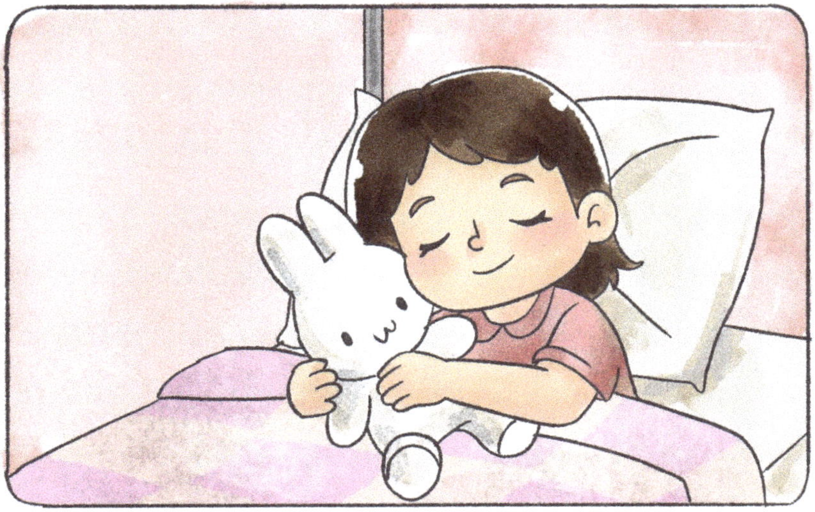

Rest helps your
body heal.

What are some things that will help you feel better?

What creative ideas do you have?

Treatments can make you feel

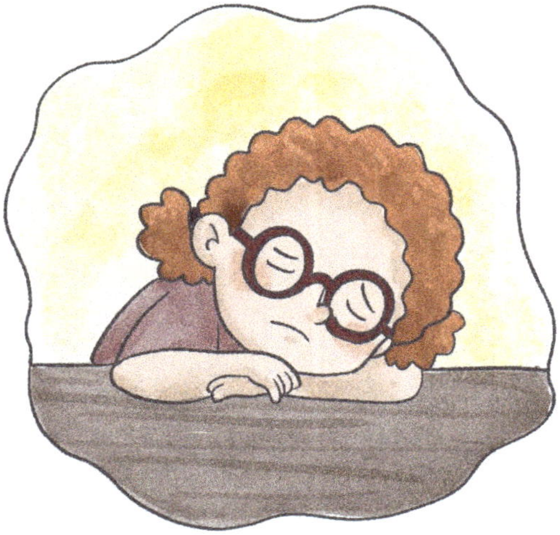

tired

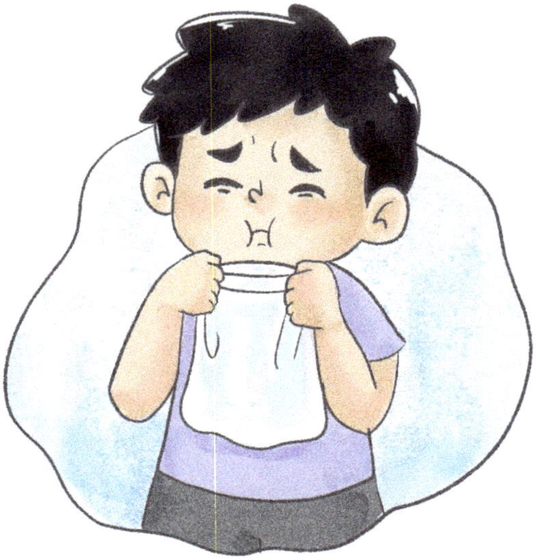

sick to your tummy

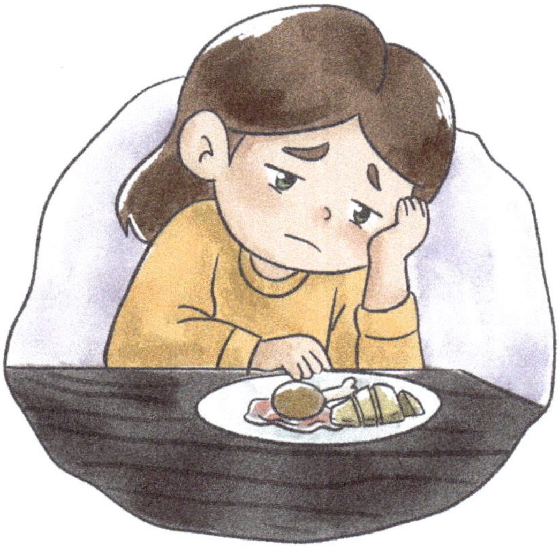

not wanting to eat much

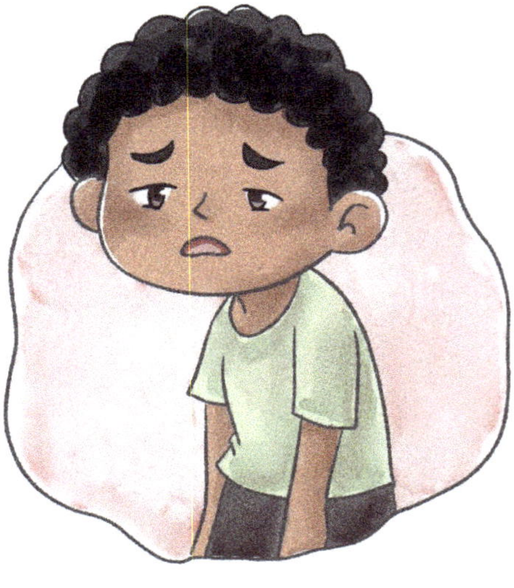

weak

Your skin may look red or feel sore.

Your hair may fall out for a little while, but it will grow back.

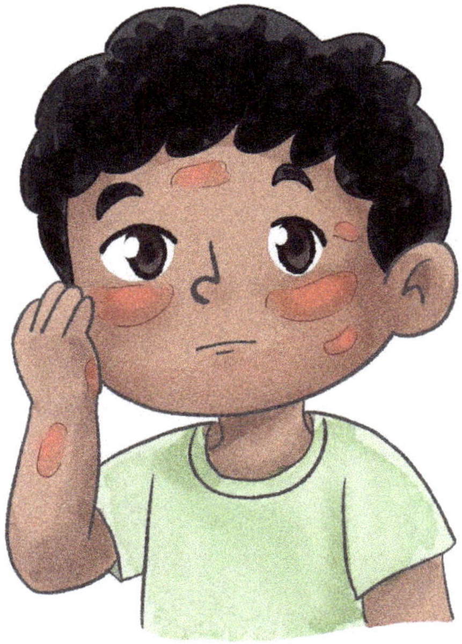

These changes mean your body is working hard and getting help.

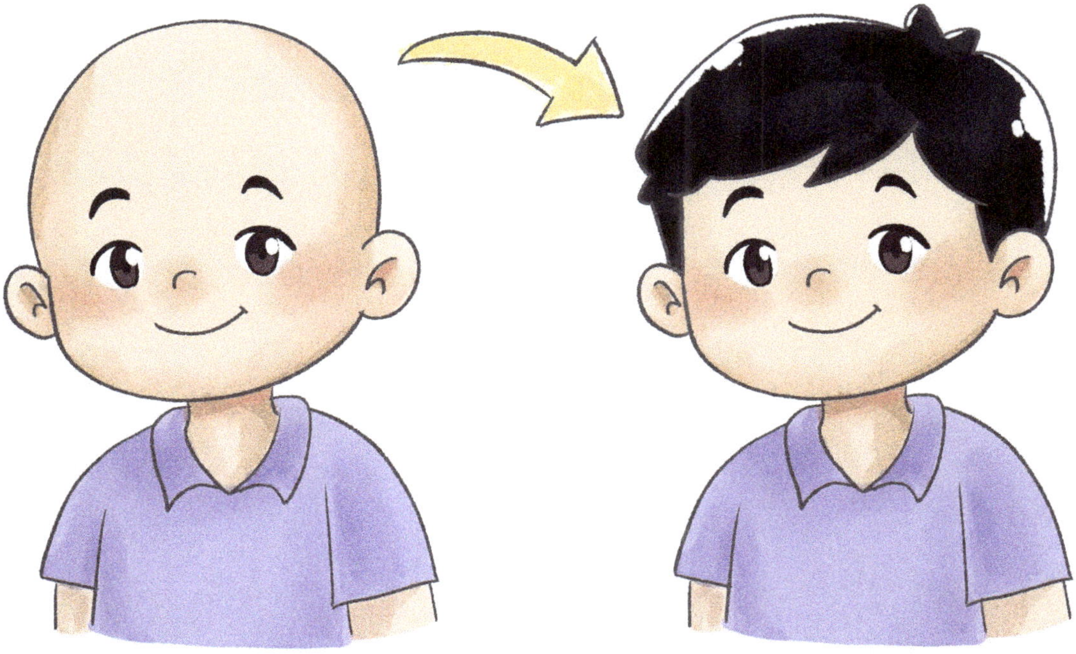

While you are healing, what would you like to do?

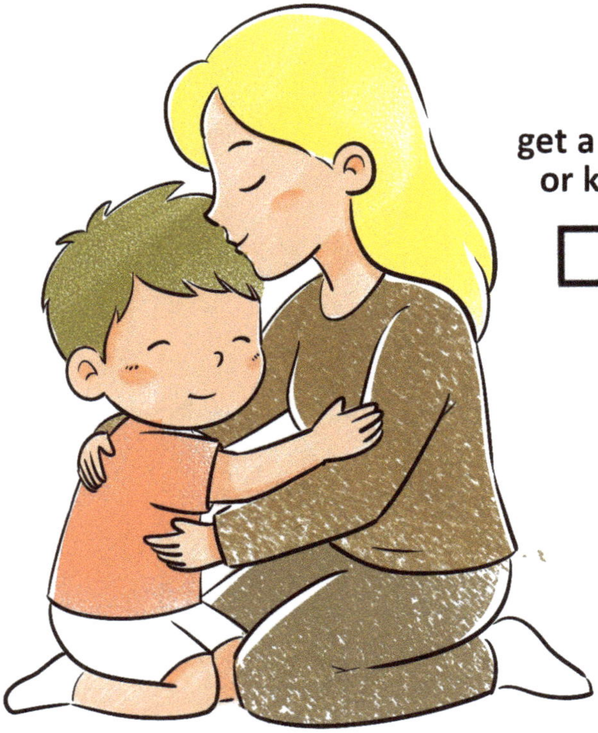

get a hug
or kiss

☐

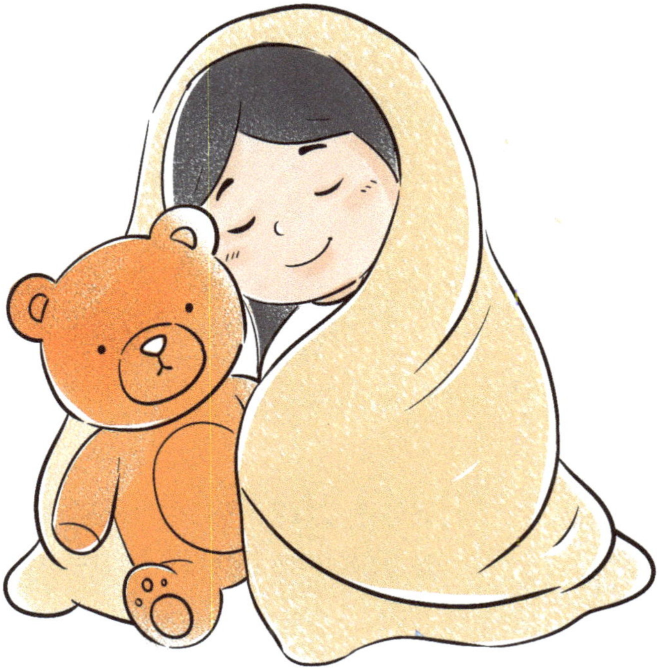

☐ rest with your favorite
blanket or toy

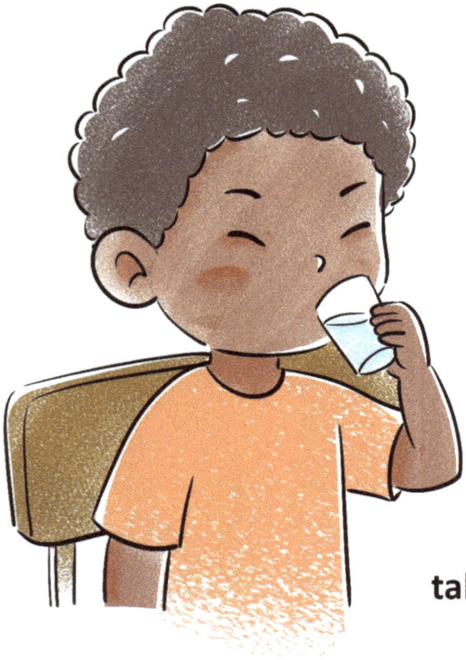

☐

take medicine

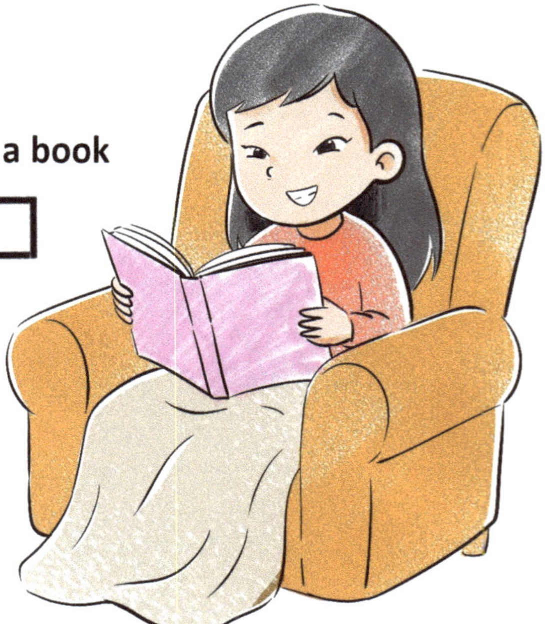

read a book

☐

☐ listen to music or a story

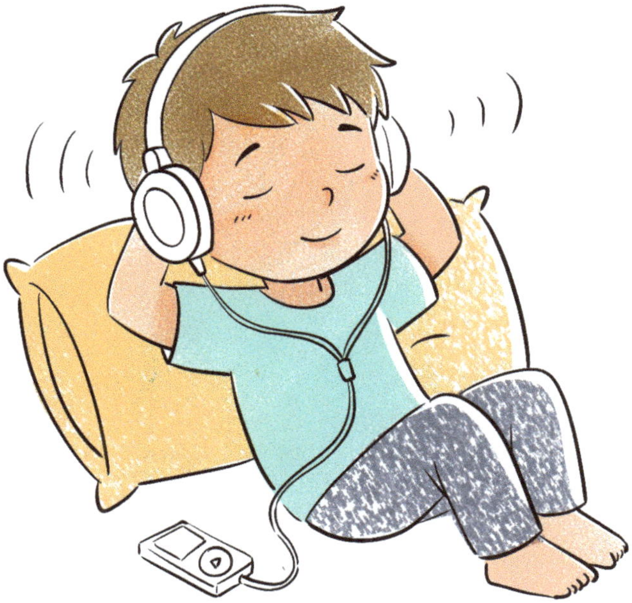

☐ watch a show

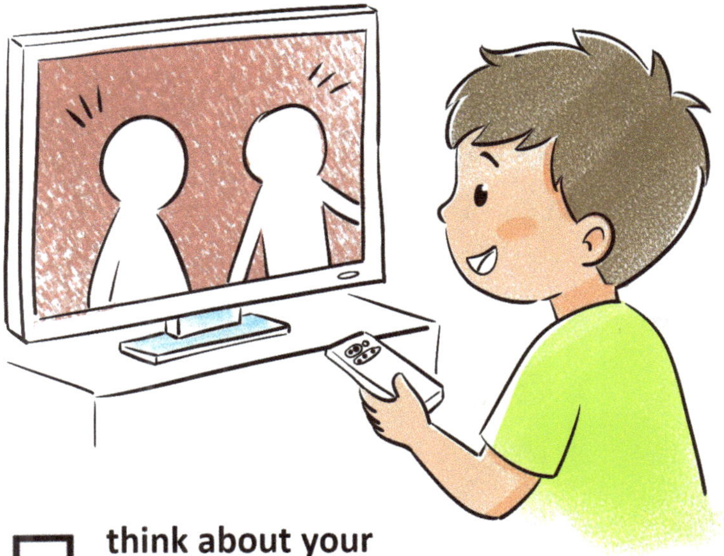

☐ think about your favorite foods

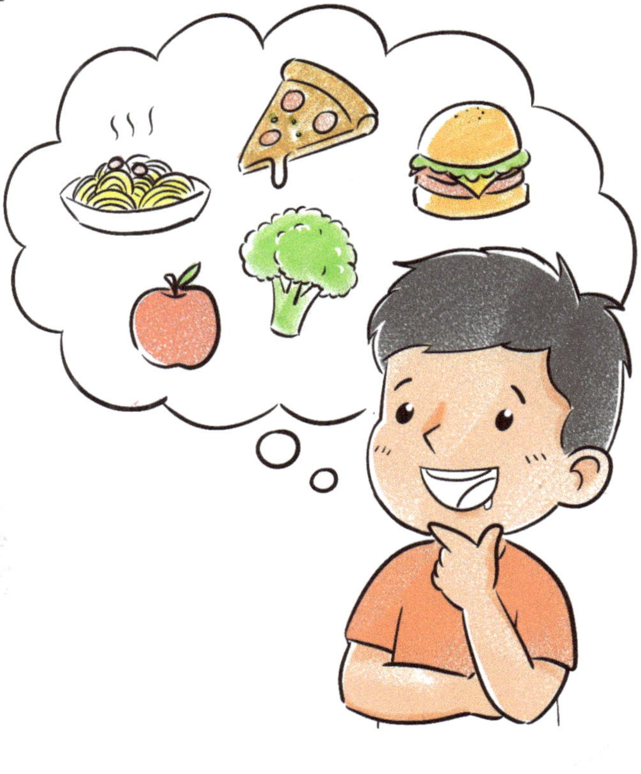

☐ draw or color

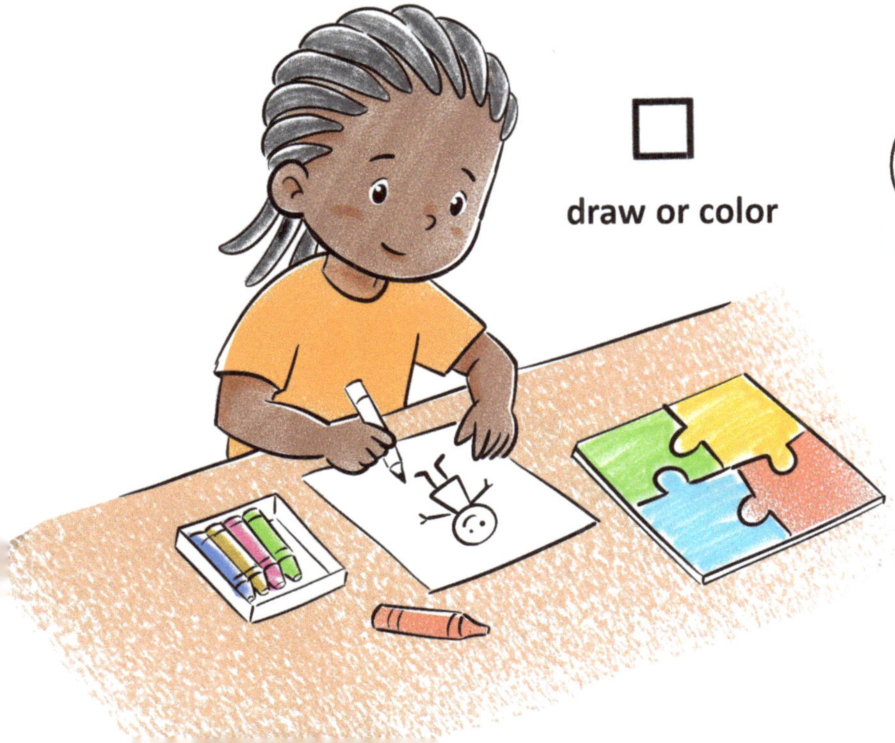

You cannot catch cancer.

You cannot give cancer to anyone.

You can still hug, cuddle, and hold hands.

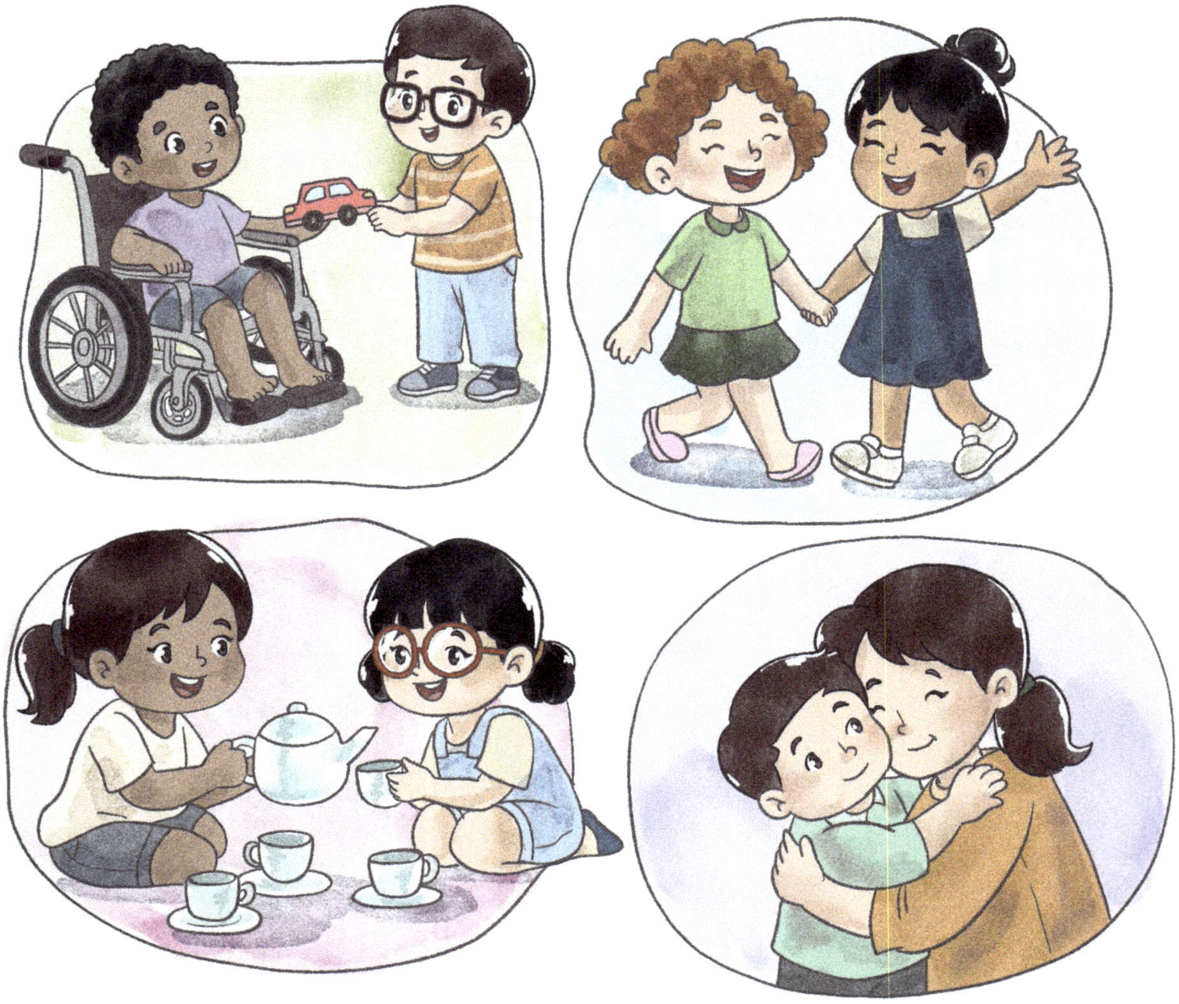

Cancer is not your fault.

You did nothing wrong.

No one can choose who gets cancer.

Things may feel different for a while,
but it will not last forever.

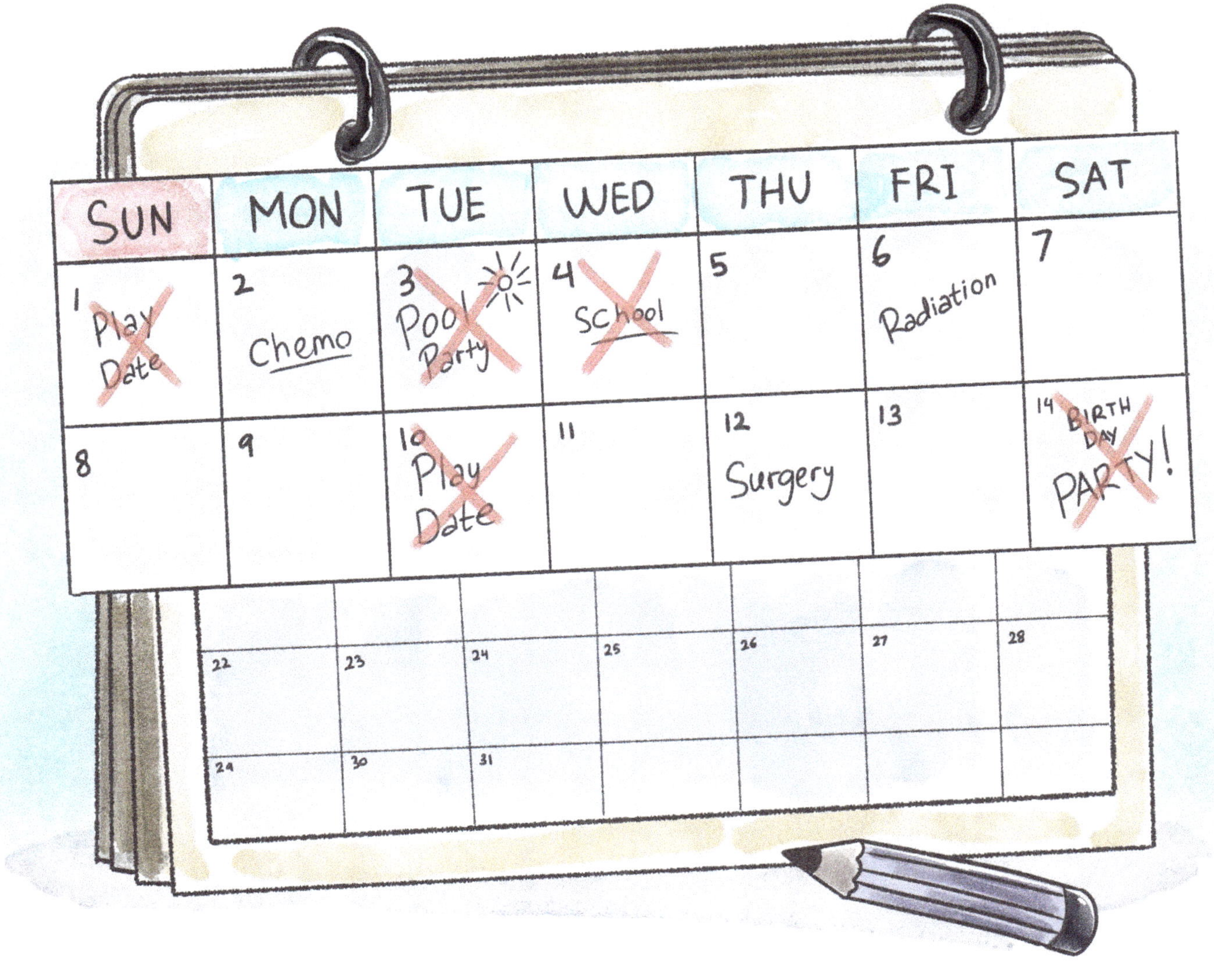

You may feel

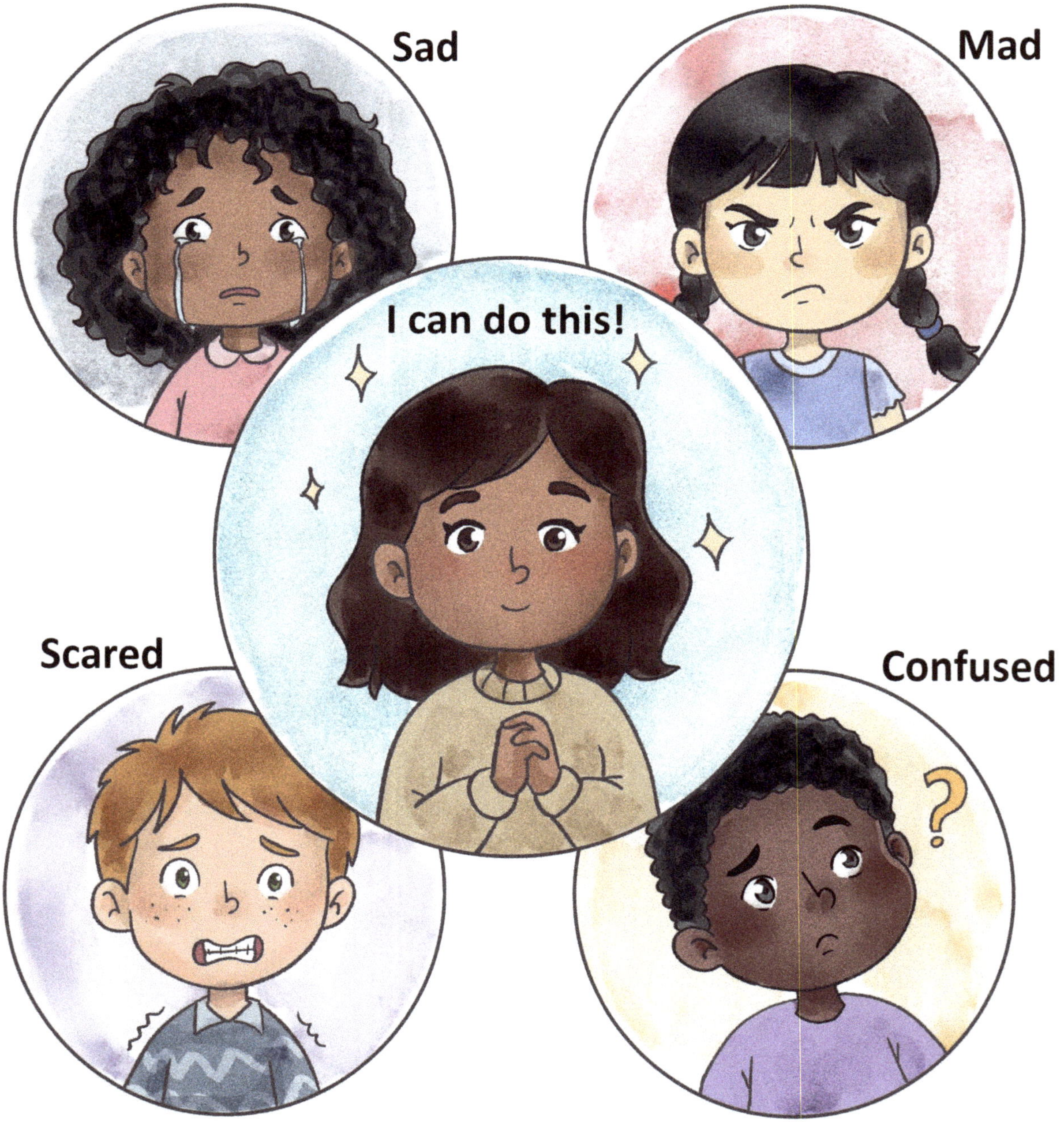

All feelings are okay.
Talking to a grown-up helps.
You can always ask questions.

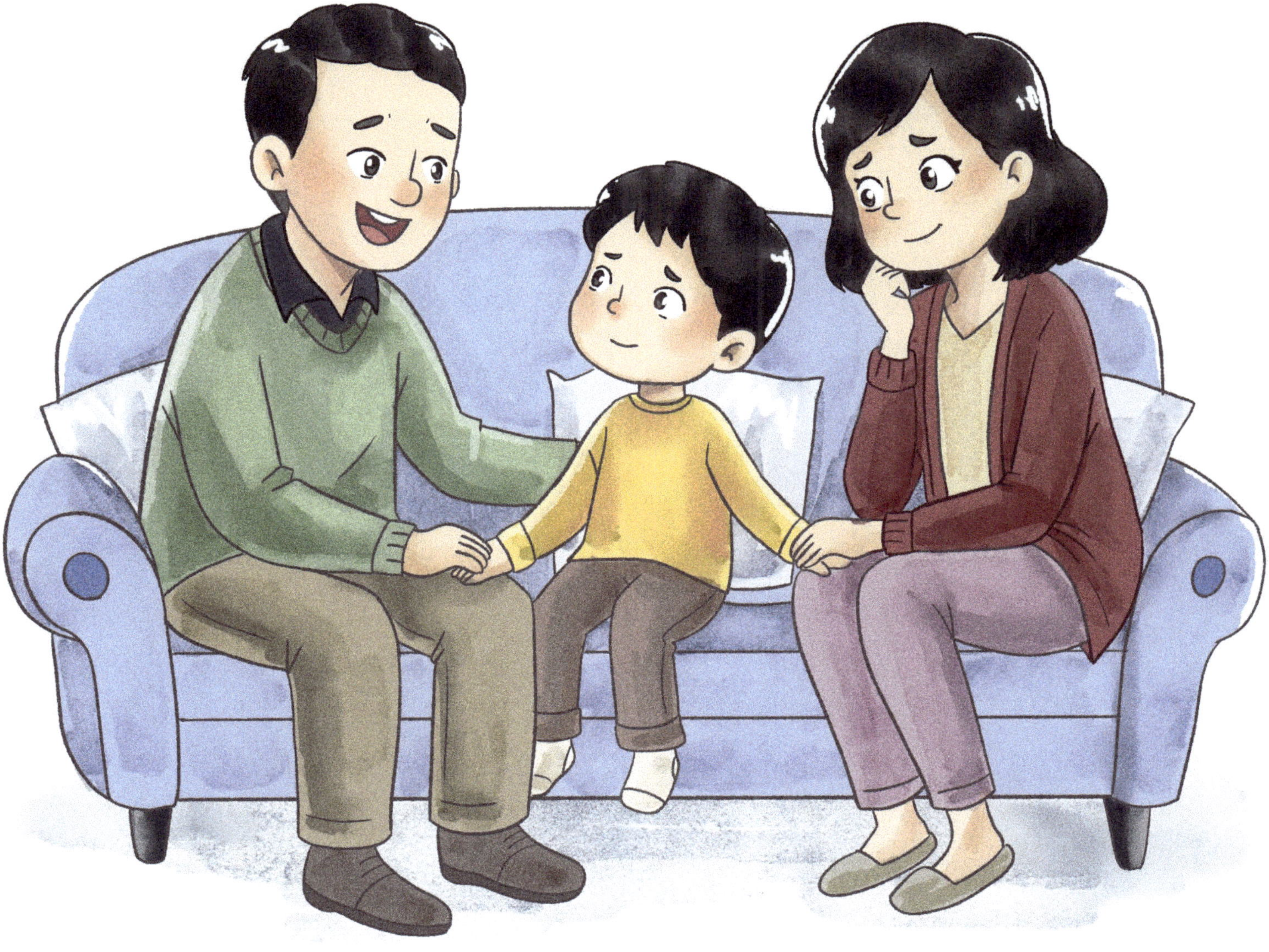

Your grown-up will stay with you.

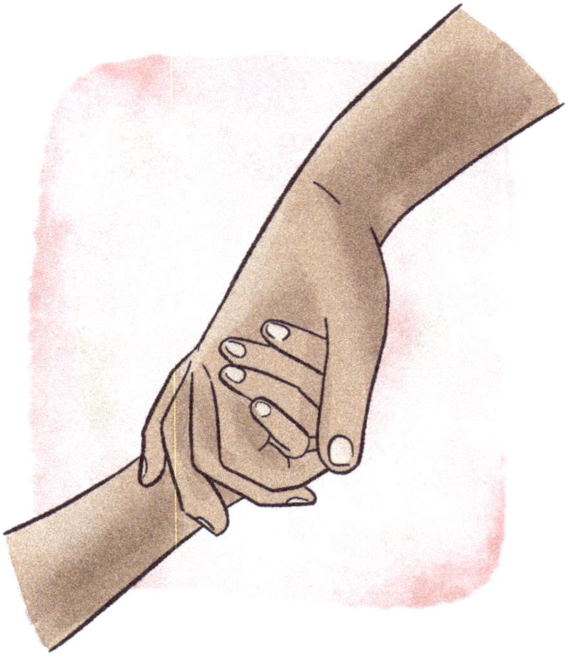

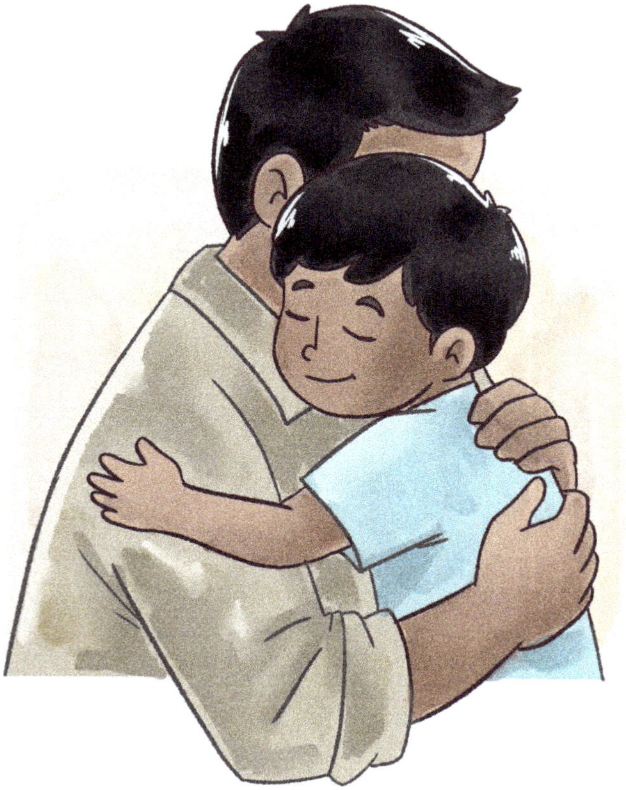

You can give hugs.

You can hold their hand.

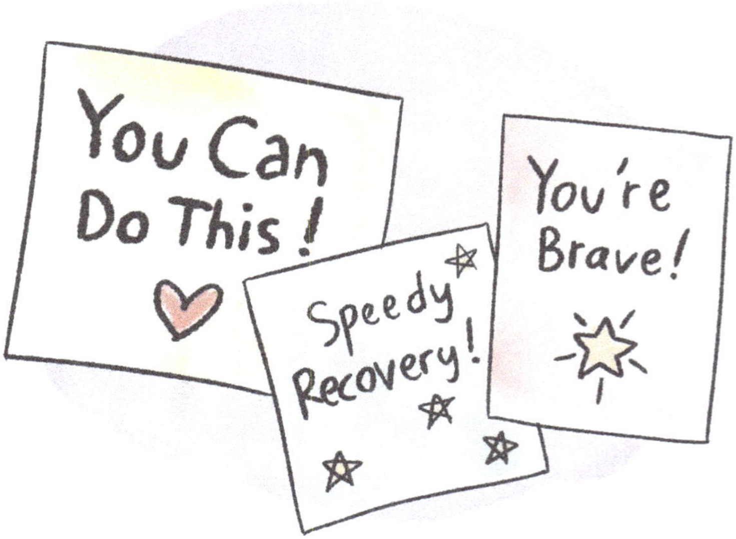

You are not alone.
You are safe.
You are loved.

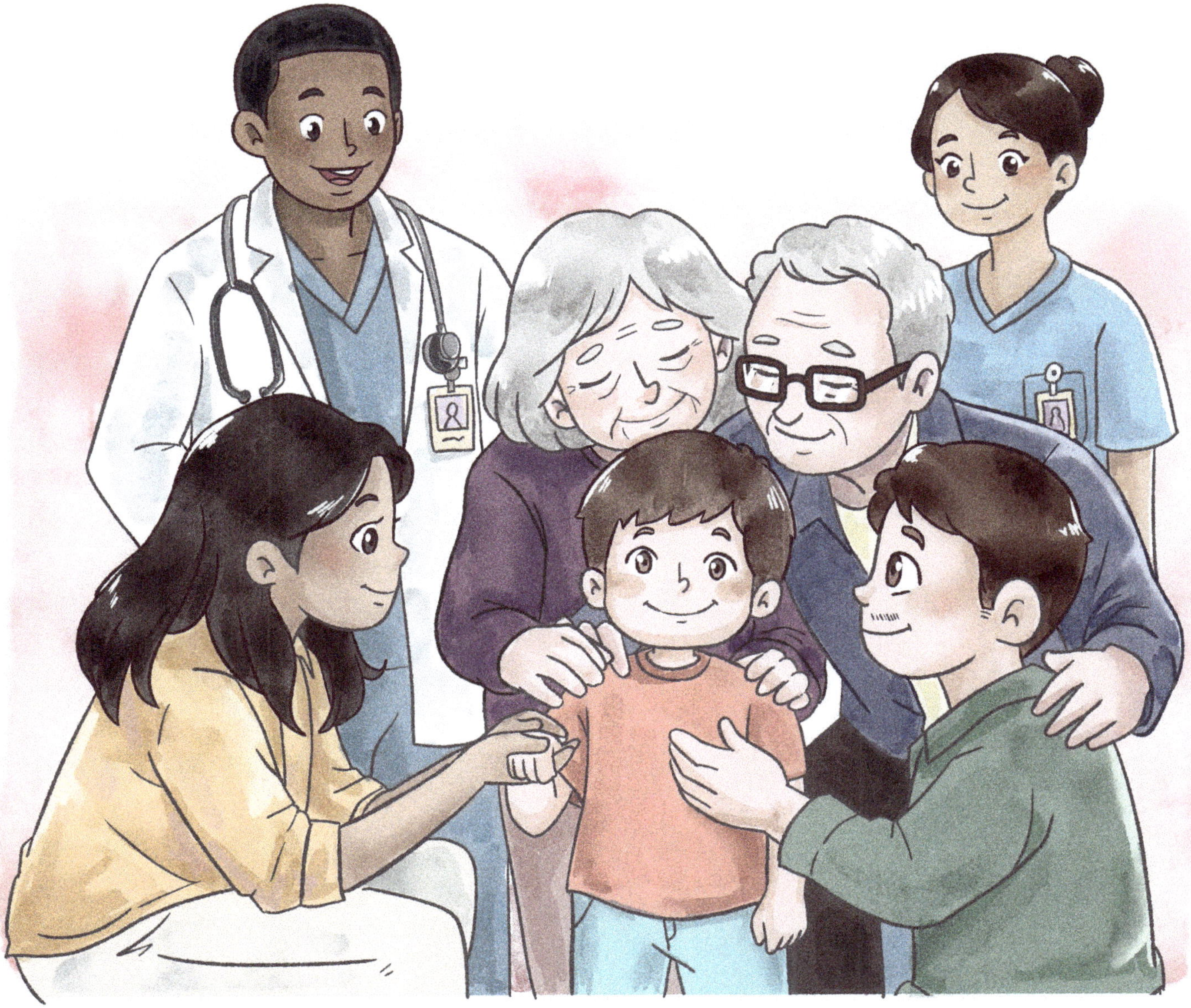

You can still play.

You can still laugh.

You can still be silly.

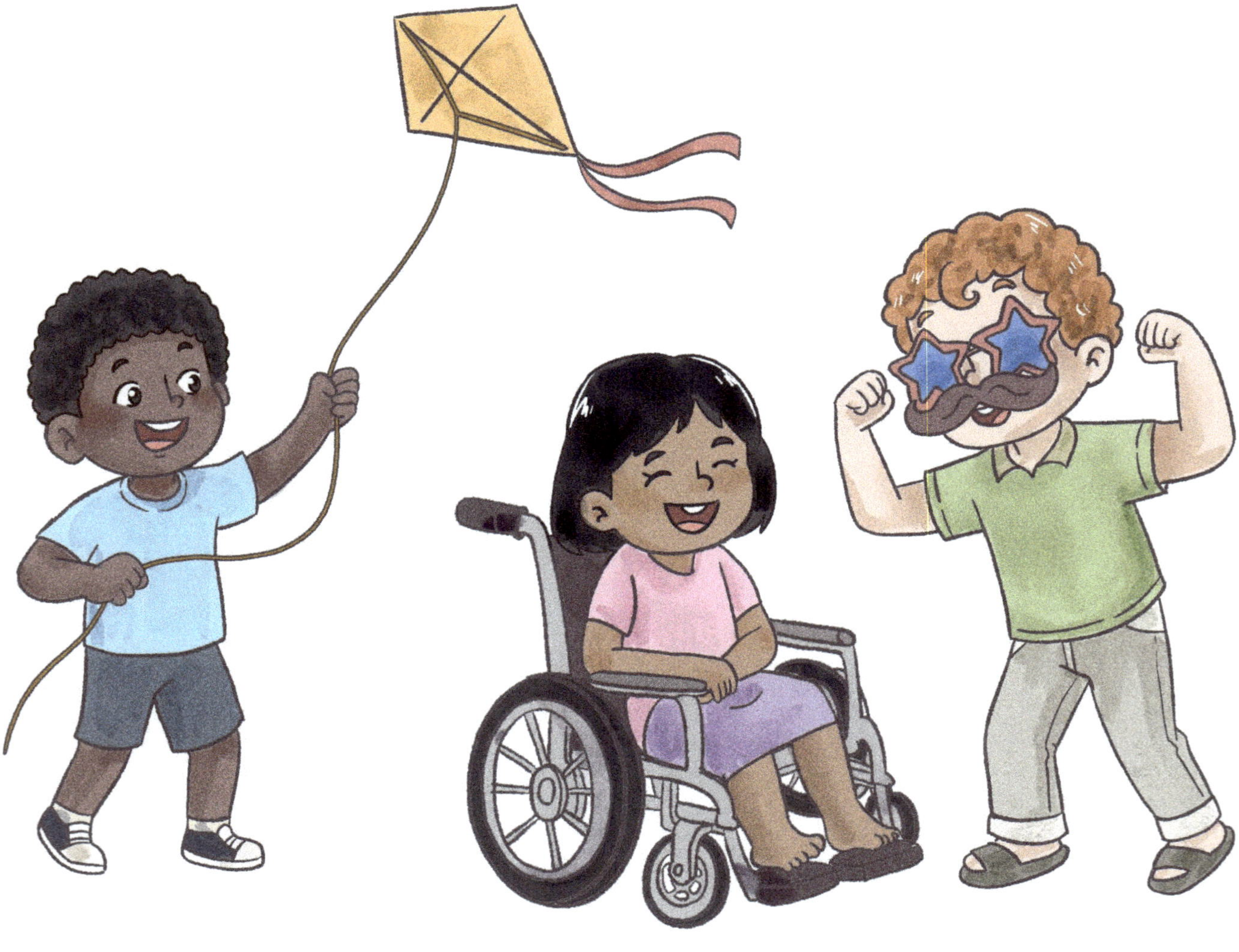

You are still brave.

You are still strong.

You are still beautiful.

And, you are doing hard things!

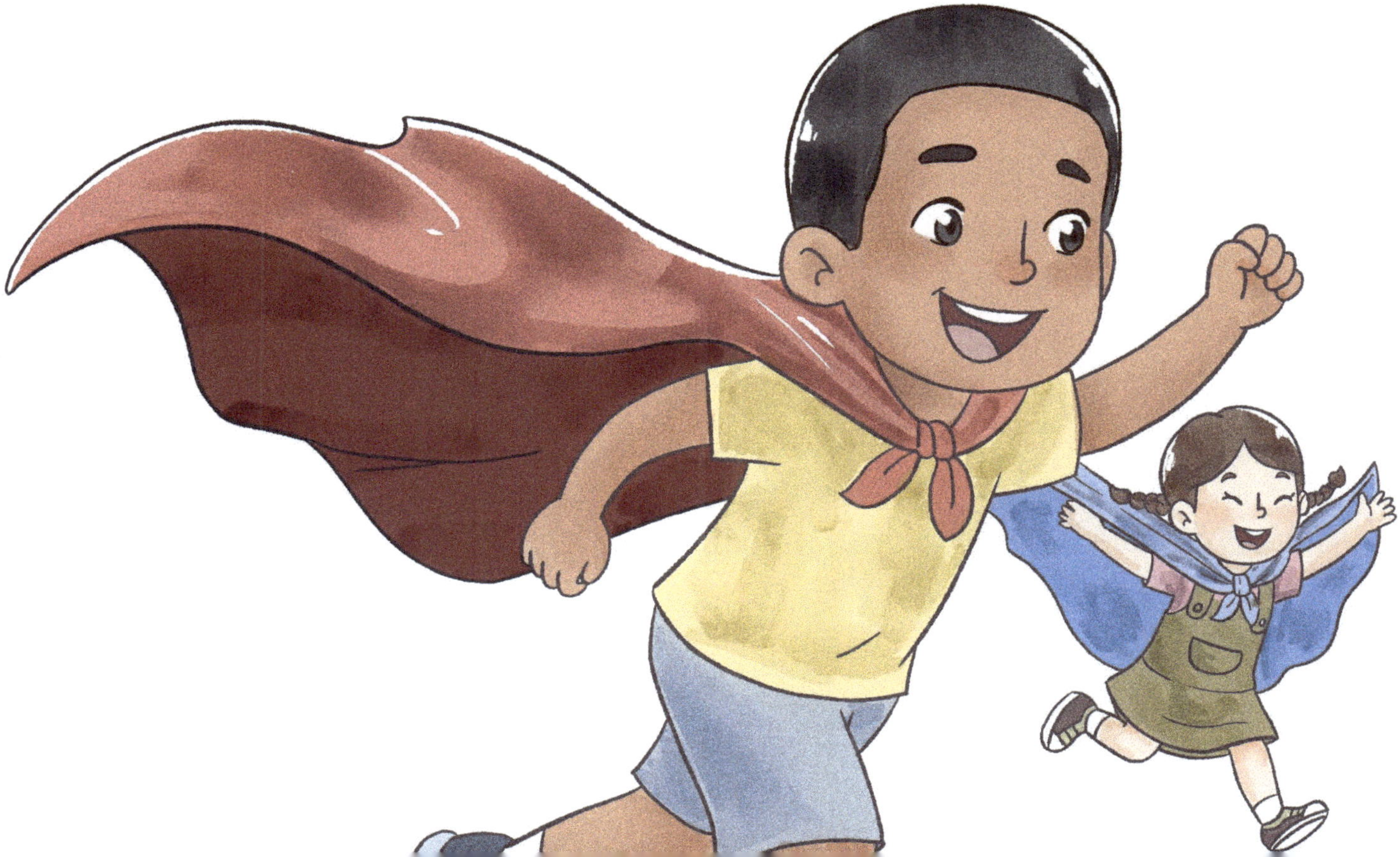

As a friend, which of the following would you like to do?
Place a checkmark (✓) next to your favorites.

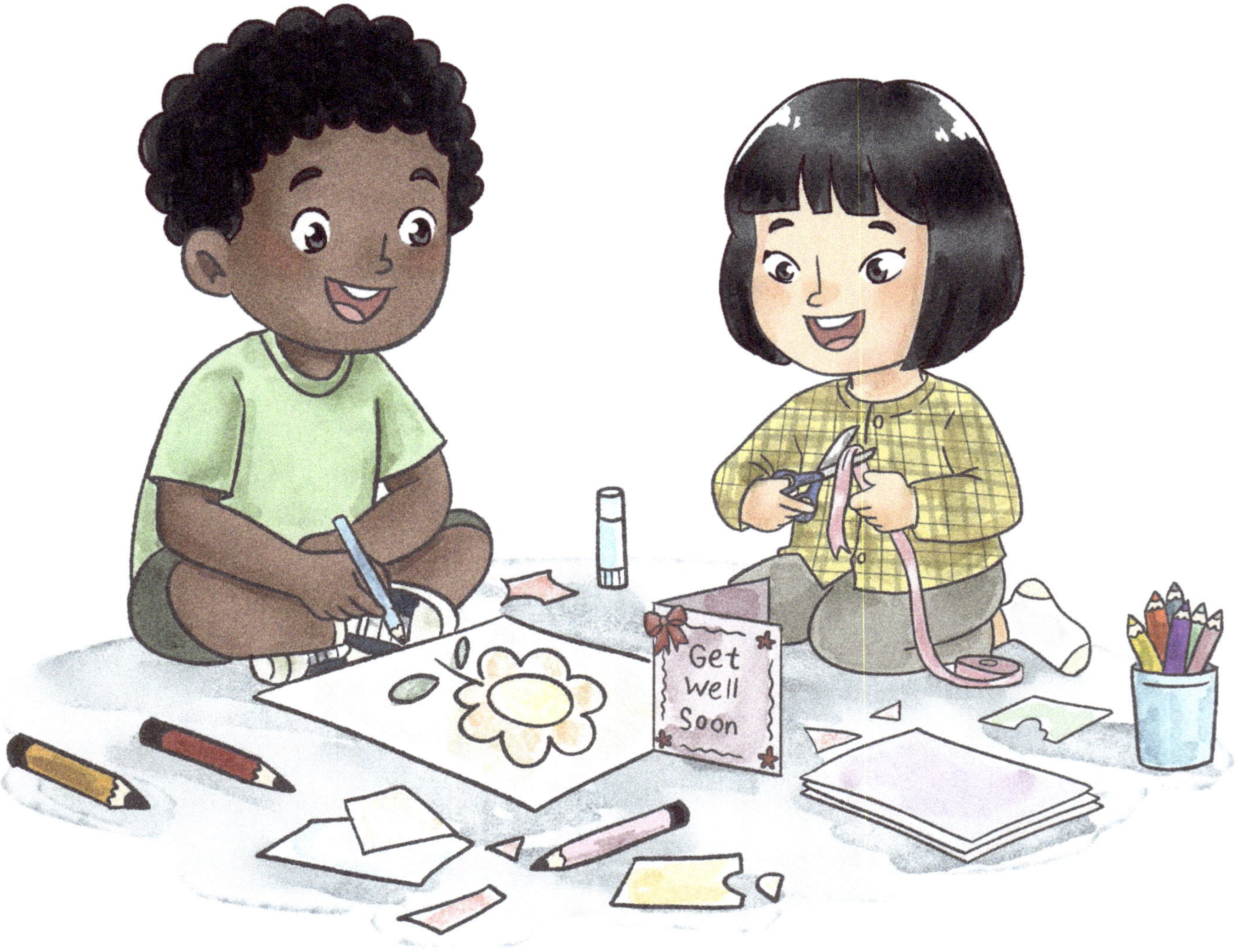

☐ Draw pictures or make cards

☐ Be patient if playtime needs to wait

☐ Wave hello on video or from far away

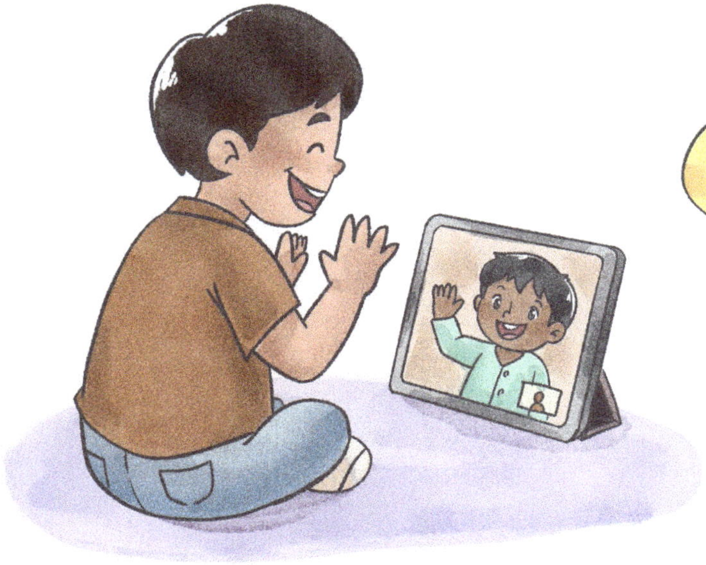

☐ Send silly jokes or kind notes

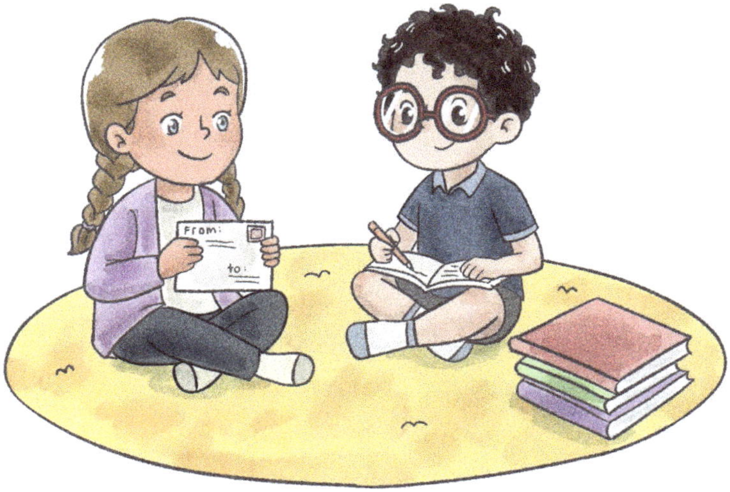

☐ Cheer them on and say, "You can do this!"

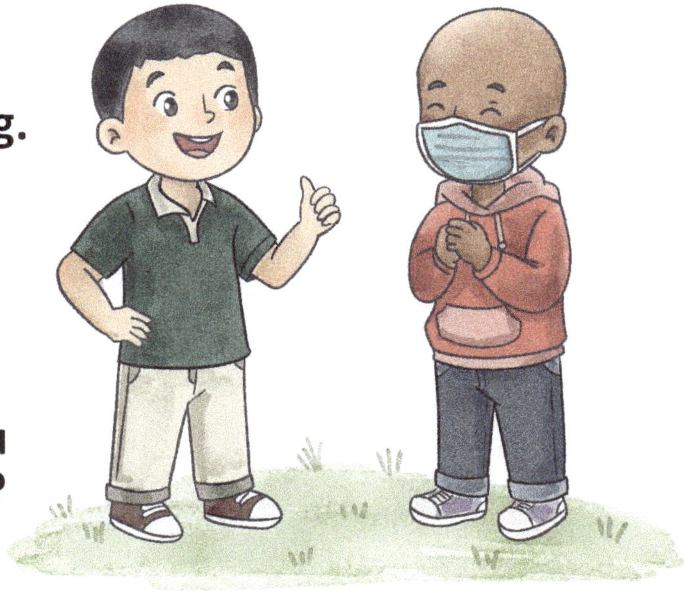

Friends don't have to fix anything.

Being kind and caring is already helping.

What are some other ways you would like to be a good friend?

Treatment takes time,

but it will not last forever.

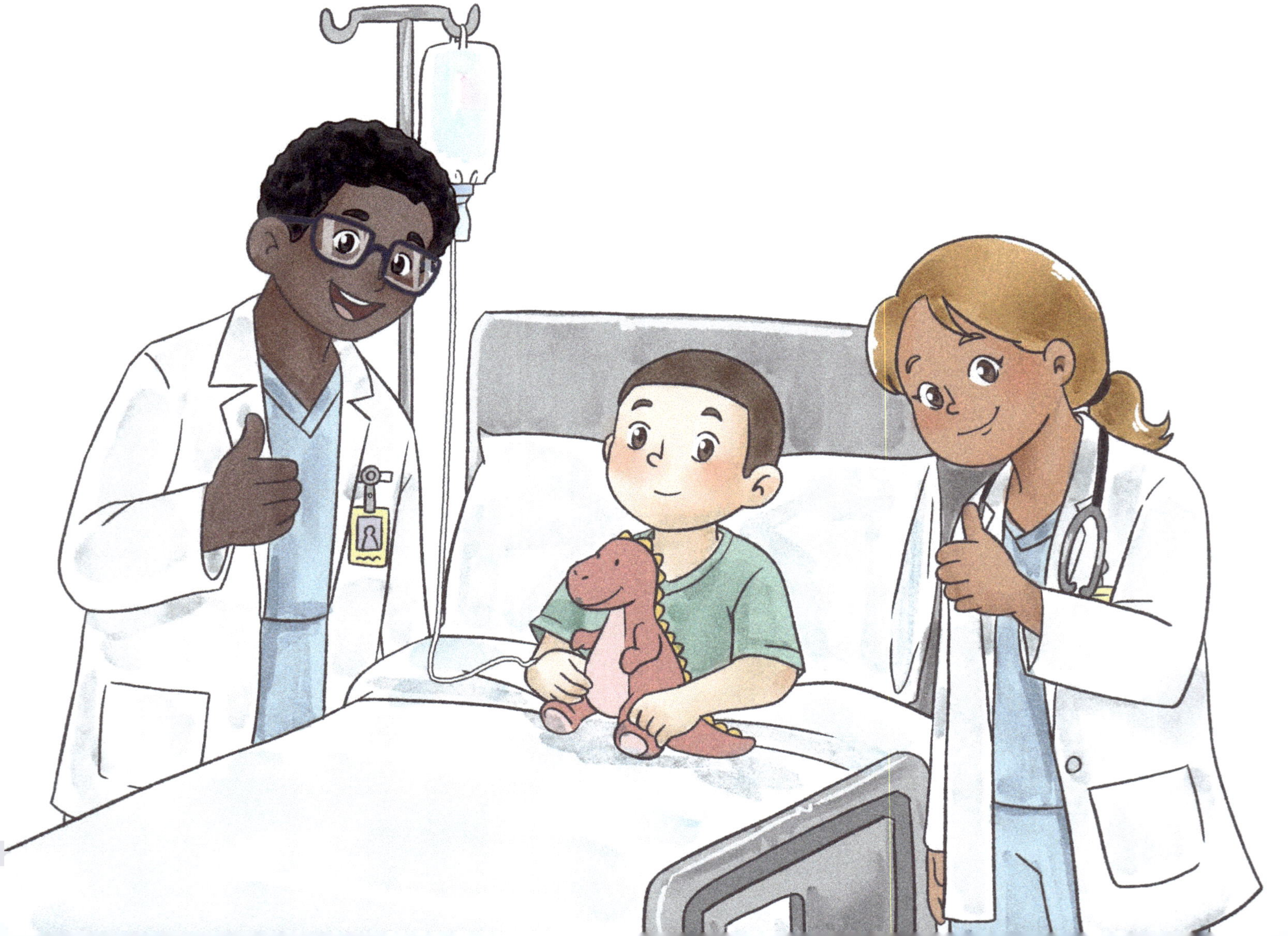

Doctors, scientists, and researchers are working hard and continue to find new ways to treat cancer.

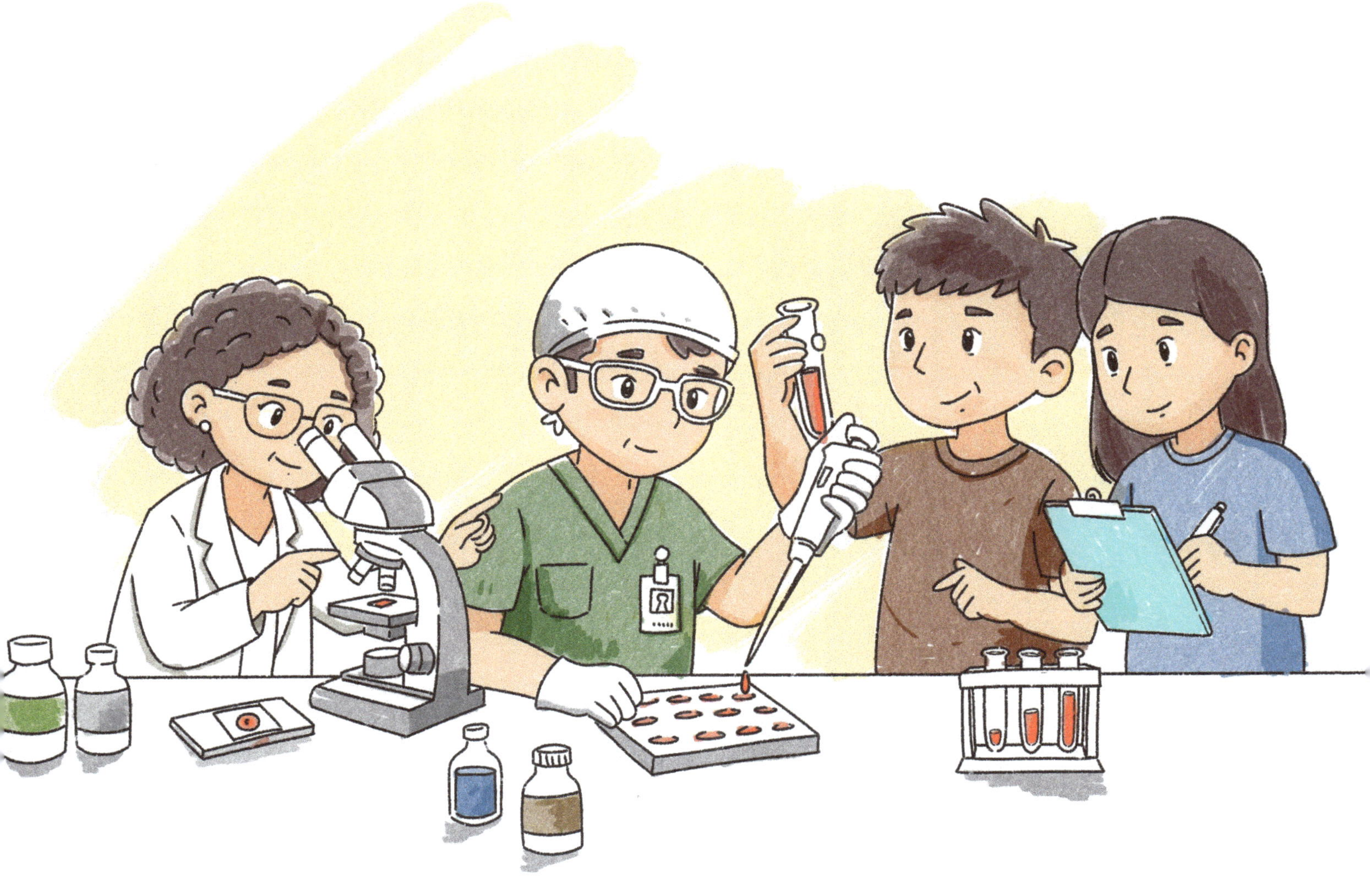

Little by little, your body can grow stronger.
Your doctor will tell you when it's time for a break from treatment or when your treatment is finished.
Many people are here to help you.

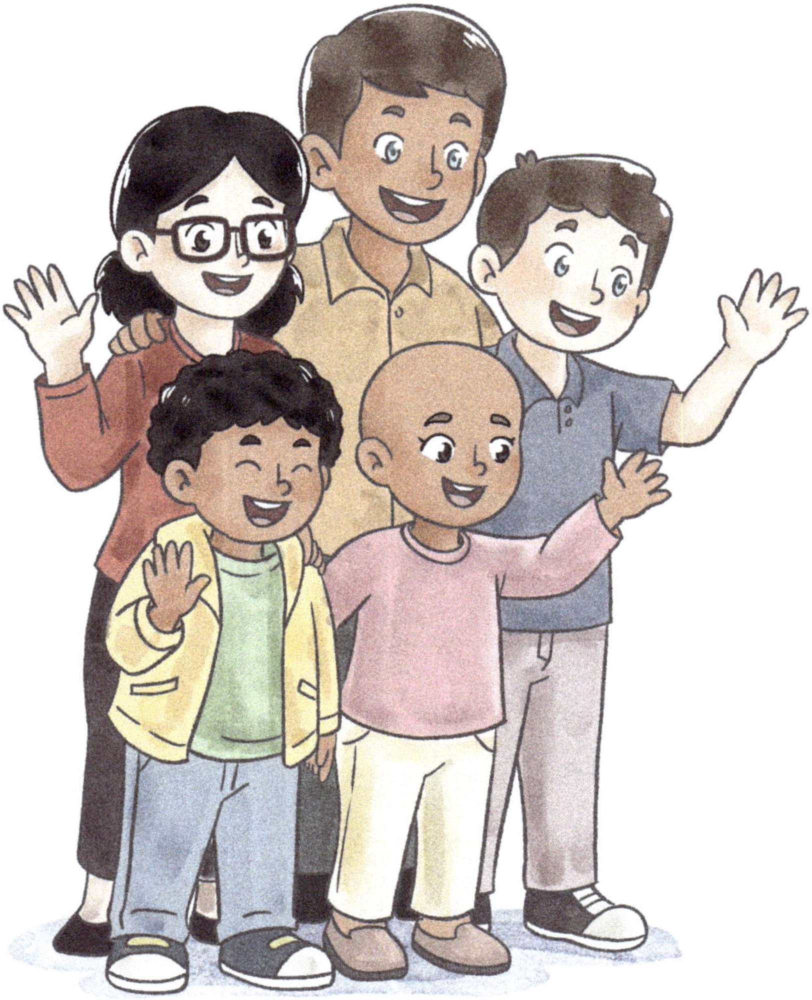

You are very loved.

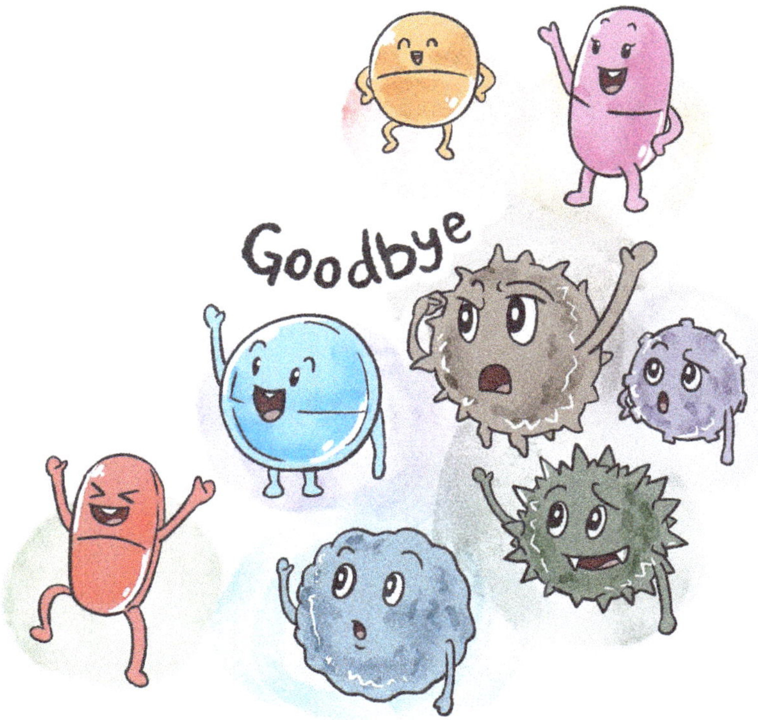
Goodbye

One day, treatment will be done.
That is a special day!

You can celebrate by:

Ringing a bell

Having a party

Eating a favorite treat

Wearing a special outfit

Taking pictures

Getting hugs and cheers

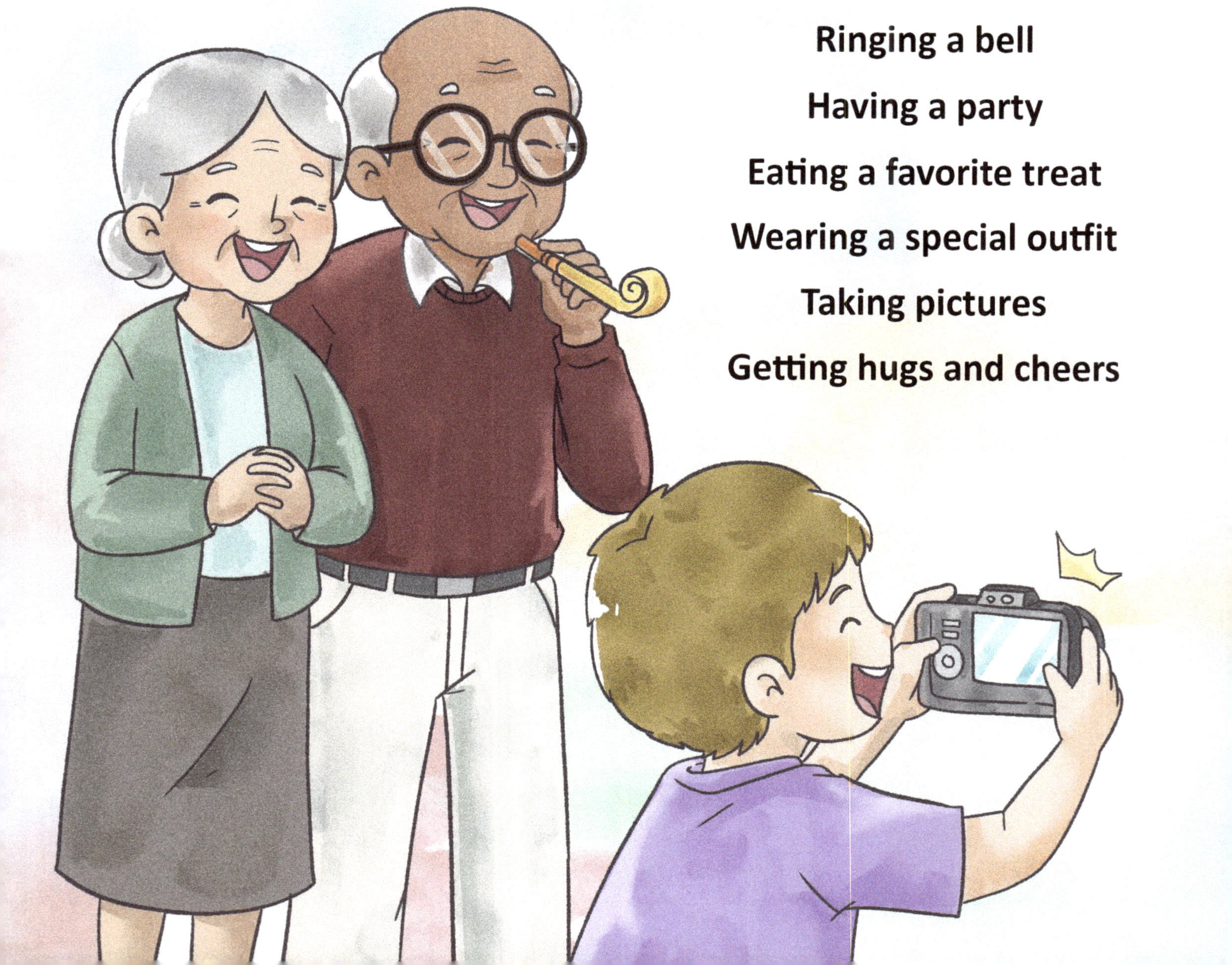

What’s your favorite way to celebrate?

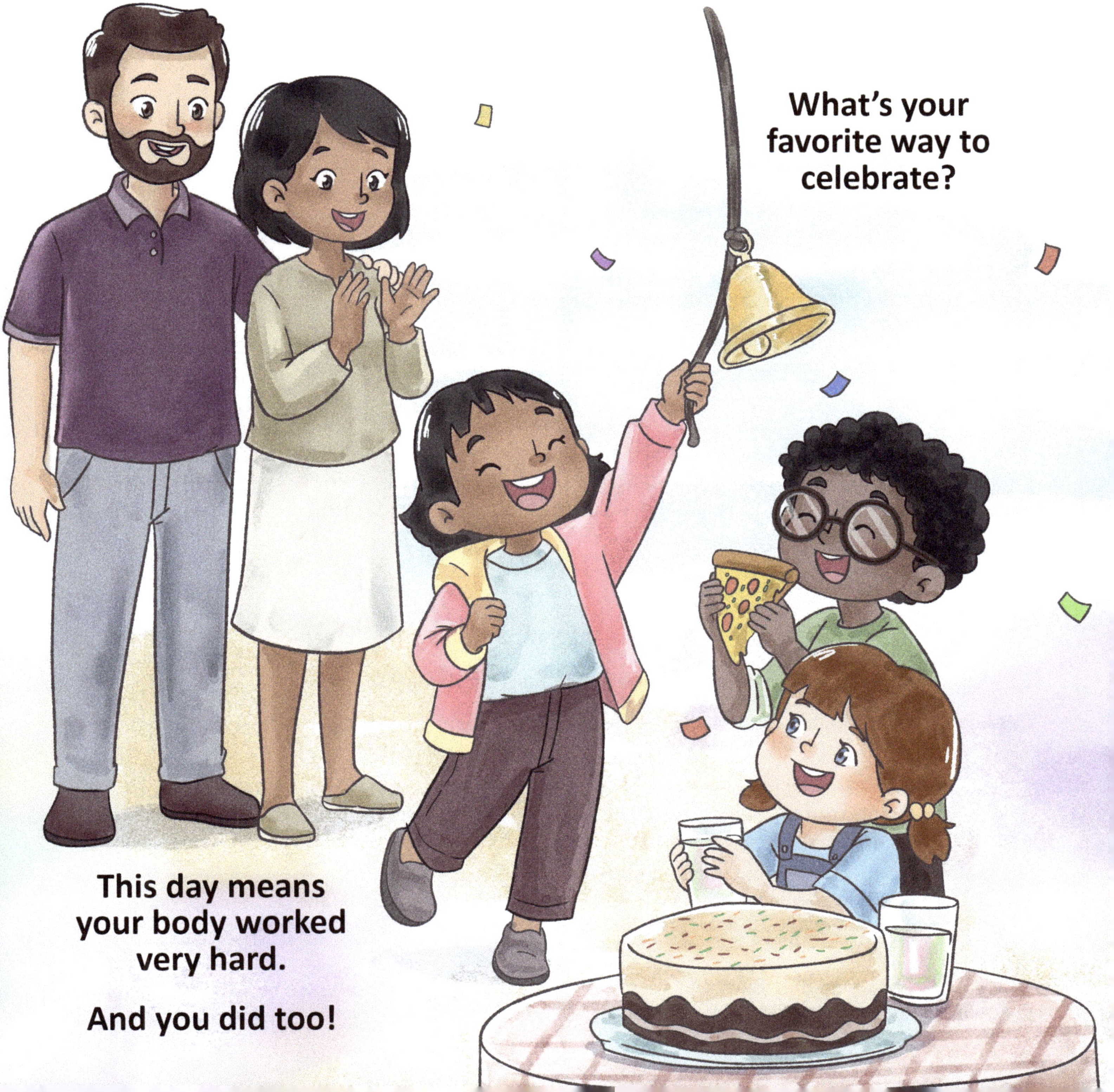

This day means your body worked very hard.

And you did too!

A Note to Parents & Caregivers

Talking to a young child about cancer can feel overwhelming. Knowing what to say—and how much to say—can be hard.

This book was created to help make those conversations gentler.

Strong Like Me: Understanding Cancer uses simple language, interactive moments, and reassuring repetition to help children understand cancer and its treatments in a calm, age-appropriate way. It also highlights how friends and loved ones can help through kindness, patience, and staying connected—because feeling supported matters just as much as understanding medical care.

You may notice repeated messages of safety and love throughout the book. These are intentional. Young children cope best with repetition, play, and the steady presence of caring adults.

Every child's experience is unique. Thus, please move through this book at your child's pace, follow their questions, and pause or revisit pages as needed. Most importantly, remind your child often that they are safe, loved, and not alone.

With care and hope,
Dr. Fei Zheng-Ward

Disclaimer

Please note that the illustrations are not drawn to scale.

This book is written for informational, educational, and personal growth purposes and should not be used as a substitute for medical advice.

Please consult your child's doctor if they need medical attention and to ensure the information in this book pertains to your child's medical condition and needs. I cannot guarantee what your child experiences is exactly what is being discussed in this book.

The author and the publisher are not responsible, either directly or indirectly, for any damages, monetary losses, or reparations due to information in this book. By reading this book, the readers agree not to hold the author and the publisher responsible for any losses as a result of any errors, inaccuracies, or omissions in this book.

Please keep in mind that your child's experience depends on the location, the facility, their medical condition, and the healthcare team. Please use this book in conjunction with your child's doctor's advice. Thank you.

Did this picture book help your child in some way?
If so, I would love to hear about it!

www.amazon.com/gp/product-review/B0HCYHFPN1

For other book titles, please visit:

www.fzwbooks.com

Connect with the author

email: books@fzwbooks.com
facebook/instagram: @FZWbooks

Books by the author

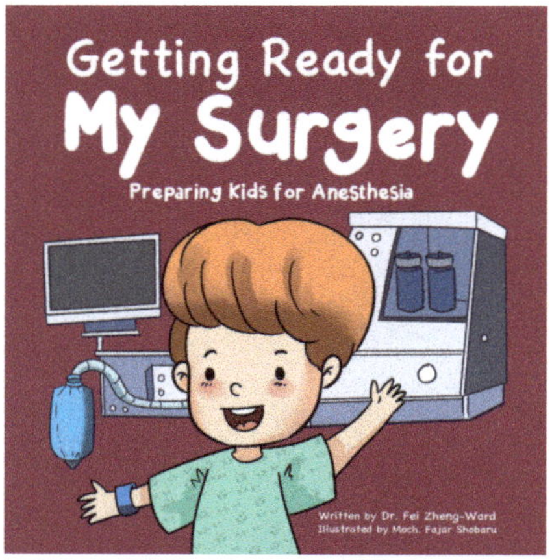

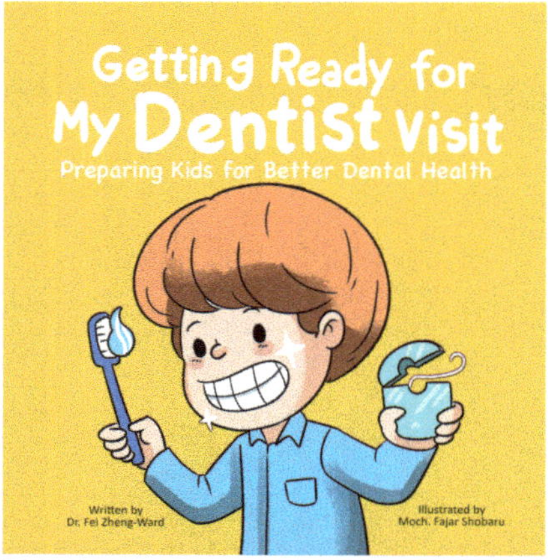

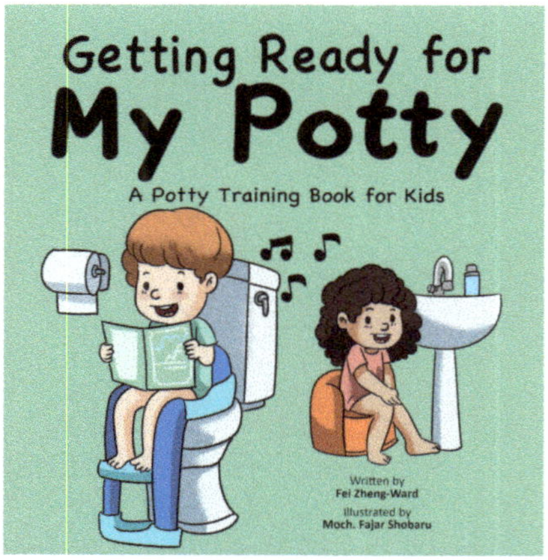

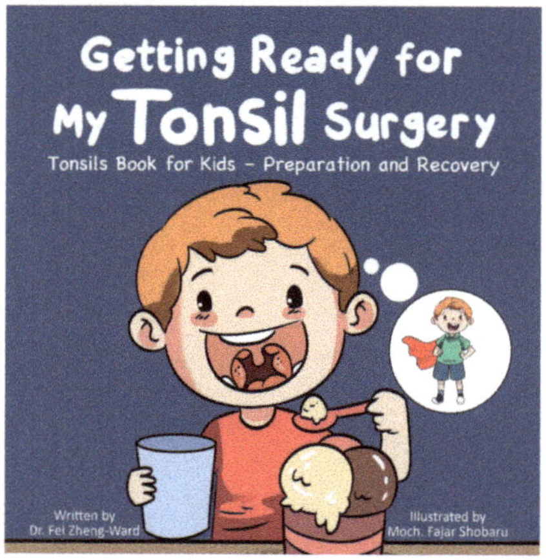

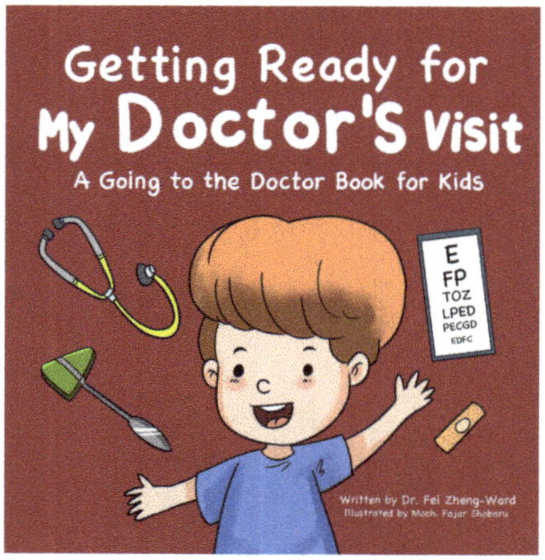

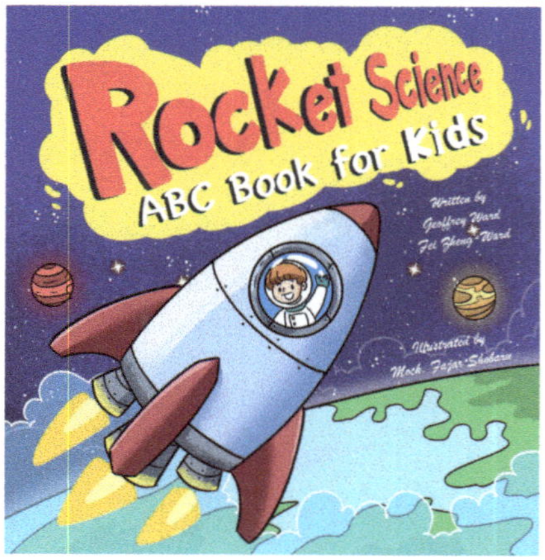

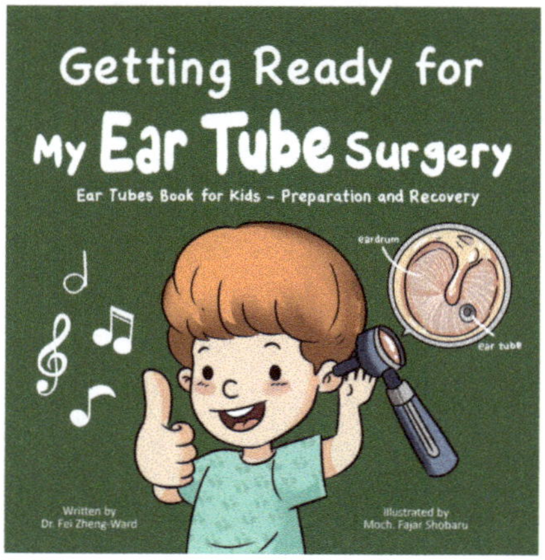

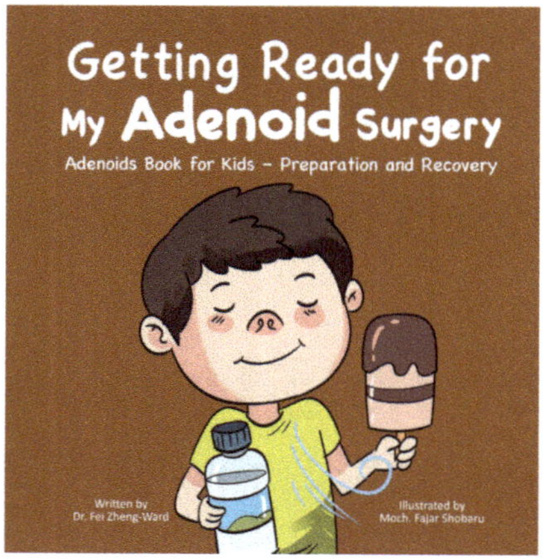

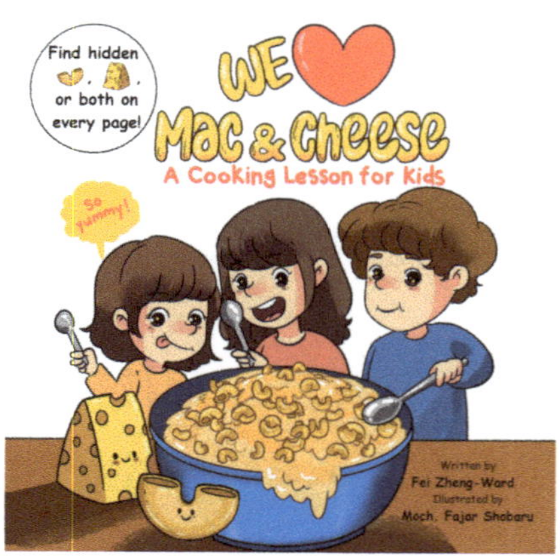

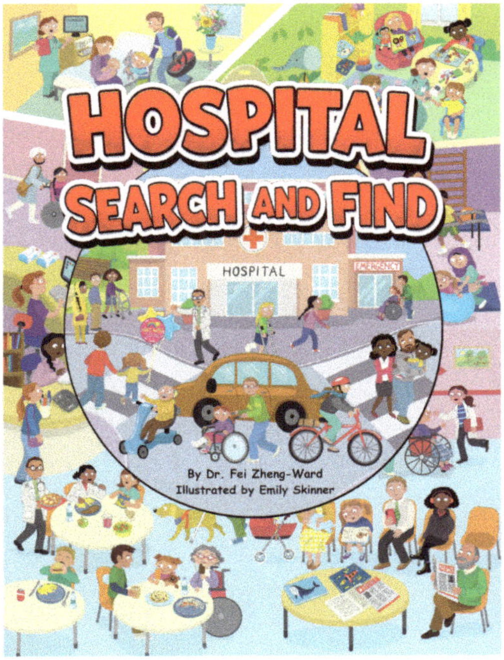
HOSPITAL
SEARCH AND FIND
HOSPITAL
By Dr. Fei Zheng-Ward
Illustrated by Emily Skinner

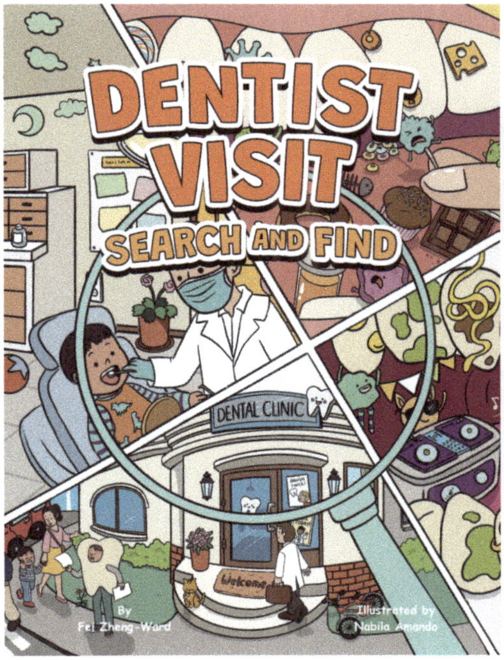
DENTIST VISIT
SEARCH AND FIND
DENTAL CLINIC
By
Fei Zheng-Ward
Illustrated by
Nabila Amanda

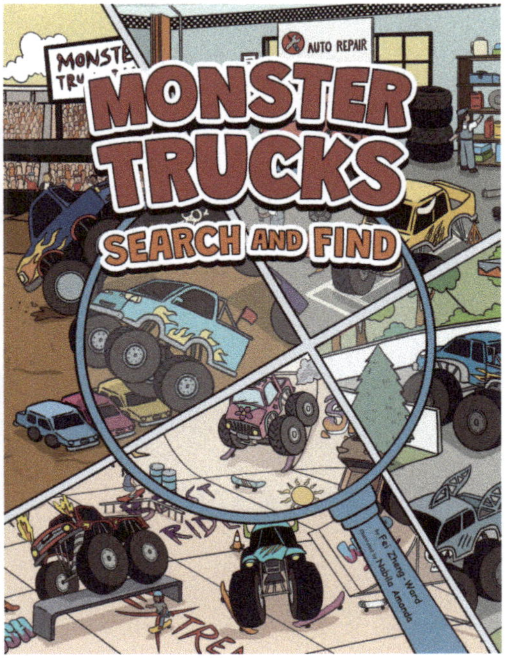
AUTO REPAIR
MONSTER TRUCKS
SEARCH AND FIND

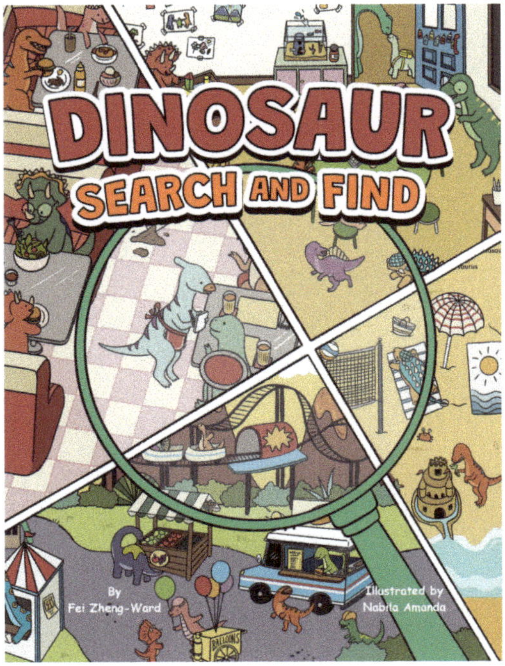
DINOSAUR
SEARCH AND FIND
By
Fei Zheng-Ward
Illustrated by
Nabila Amanda

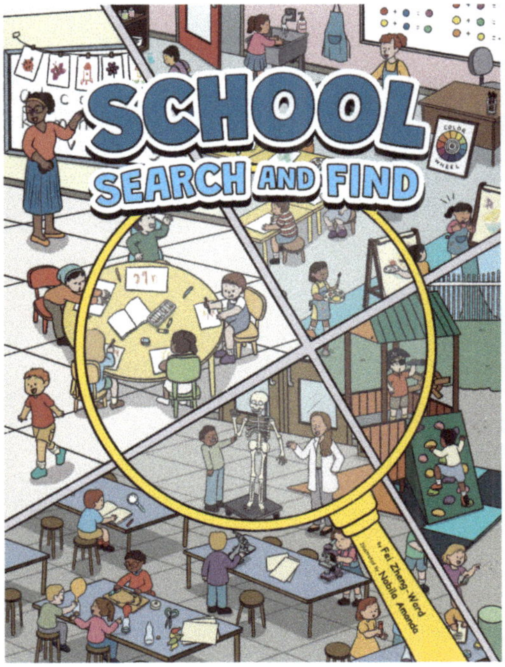
SCHOOL
SEARCH AND FIND

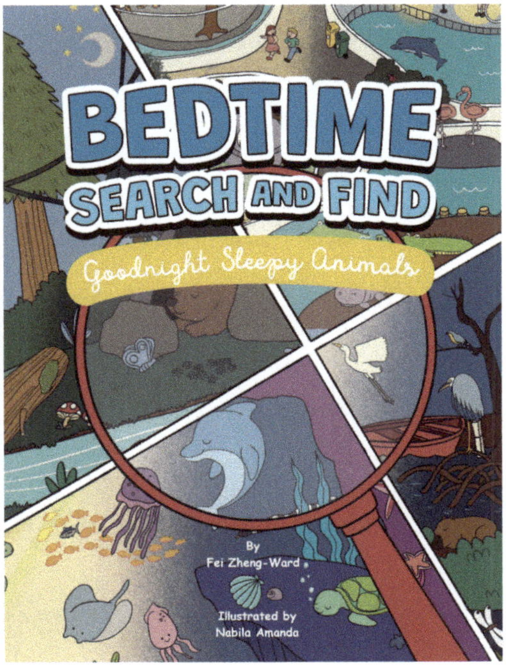
BEDTIME
SEARCH AND FIND
Goodnight Sleepy Animals
By
Fei Zheng-Ward
Illustrated by
Nabila Amanda

www.ingramcontent.com/pod-product-compliance
Lightning Source LLC
LaVergne TN
LVHW070444061126
851858LV00011B/157
9798893181463